Masuda

TELEMEDICINE AND THE REINVENTION OF HEALTHCARE

TELEMEDICINE AND THE REINVENTION OF HEALTHCARE

JEFFREY BAUER

MARC RINGEL

McGraw-Hill

New York   San Francisco   Washington, D.C.   Auckland   Bogotá
Caracas   Lisbon   London   Madrid   Mexico City   Milan
Montreal   New Delhi   San Juan   Singapore
Sydney   Tokyo   Toronto

McGraw-Hill

A Division of The **McGraw·Hill** Companies

1 2 3 4 5 6 7 8 9 0 BKM/BKM 9 0 9 8 7

ISBN 007-134630-9

Printing and binding by Book-Mart Press, Inc.

Cover illustration by Steve Dininno.

This book was typeset using 10 point Times Roman.

This publication is designed to provide accurate and authoritative information in regard to the subject matter covered. It is sold with the understanding that neither the author nor the publisher is engaged in rendering legal, accounting, or other professional service. If legal advice or other expert assistance is required, the services of a competent professional person should be sought.

> —*From a Declaration of Principles jointly adopted by a Committee of the American Bar Association and a Committee of Publishers.*

C O N T E N T S

1

CHAPTER

Introduction

Telemedicine, one of the major forces shaping the future of healthcare, is widely misunderstood. Its long-term impact on healthcare is obscured by excessive concerns with short-term policy problems, a misleading focus on narrow definitions, or utopian expectations of technology. People who overreact to telemedicine's early difficulties or underestimate its scope will be surprised by its real power. Telemedicine will ultimately revolutionize healthcare—restructuring virtually every relationship and activity that define late twentieth century medicine.

This book is written to bridge the gap between today's misconceptions about telemedicine and the reality of an entire industry being transformed by information sciences, communications, and computer technologies. The following chapters, interviews, and boxes are assembled for the specific purpose of exploring how clinical practice is being changed by the technologies that collectively make telemedicine possible.

However, this book is not technically oriented. Many manuals and periodicals already exist to help clinicians or managers who need to have an operational understanding of the difference between ISDN and DSL or LAN and LATA. The glossary in Chapter 9 provides definitions of technical terms for readers who want to devote extra time to becoming proficient in the advanced language of telemedicine.

Annotated references in Chapter 8 will also direct interested readers to applied technical detail.

By avoiding technical concepts in the main text, this book is suitable for anyone interested in the emerging foundations of healthcare in the twenty-first century. It is written in nontechnical English for health professionals, consumers, policymakers, and all others who want to understand the meaning of telemedicine without needing to know how to configure a system or connect cables. To borrow a metaphor from music (an important avocation for both authors), the approach here is equivalent to a music appreciation class for people who want to understand and enjoy the concert; it is not a method book full of scales and exercises for musicians who want to be in the orchestra.

This work also combines the complementary perspectives of a health futurist/medical economist (Bauer) who studies the trends in healthcare to forecast the future and a practicing family doctor/radio commentator (Ringel) who has personally spent many years using information sciences to enhance the delivery of healthcare. If some topics compel joint authorship, telemedicine is surely one of them. Neither the future-focused analyst nor the pragmatic practitioner could do full justice to this subject from a single perspective. Synthesis is essential to understanding this revolution in medicine. Our collaboration mirrors the multiple dimensions of telemedicine, so two authors are better than one on this expansive topic.

What, then, is telemedicine? And why does it matter?

HISTORICAL DEFINITIONS OF TELEMEDICINE

Telemedicine has been an evolutionary concept since the term became common in the early 1990s. The origin of the term is most often traced to 1968, when a group of physicians created a video link between Massachusetts General Hospital and Logan Airport in Boston.[1] Originally intended to support consultations for passengers who required emergency care, the system was soon being used to provide some basic health services to airport employees.

However, earlier working examples of the concept are cited in some other published sources.[2]

- In 1959, the Nebraska Psychiatric Institute installed a two-way microwave video link between the Department of Psychiatry at the University of Nebraska Medical School in Omaha and the state mental hospital in Norfolk. The system was used for neurological consultations, education, and administrative functions.

- The Space Technology Applied to Rural Papago Advanced Health Care (STARPAHC) program used technologies developed by the National Aeronautics and Space Administration (NASA) and Lockheed to establish communications between a Public Health Service hospital and a mobile examining room on the Papago Indian Reservation in Arizona during the late 1950s.
- At about the same time, Dartmouth Medical School developed and installed its Interact system to link the teaching hospital in Hanover, New Hampshire, with healthcare providers in eight outlying rural communities. Medical consultations and some allied health services were provided over this microwave link for a few years.

Several different definitions have been advanced in print and everyday usage, and no single meaning has clearly predominated. Here are a few typical definitions that illustrate the field's meaning over the past few years, arranged in sequence by year of publication to demonstrate that the compass of telemedicine has been expanding. Telemedicine is:

> . . . a system of healthcare delivery in which physicians examine distant patients through the use of telecommunications technology.[3]
> . . . the use of telecommunications for medical diagnosis and patient care.[4]
> . . . the use of telecommunications and information technology to provide healthcare services to persons who are at some distance from the provider.[5]
> . . . new uses of information and technologies [that] are emerging, as well as the ability to move the caregiver and information to where the patient is rather than moving the patient to centralized places to deliver health services and information. Today's telemedicine model is evolving to "teleconsultation," where a physician consults with other specialists or a patient, using high-quality videoconferencing, with that consultation enabled by online information access.[6]
> . . . remote communication of information to facilitate clinical care and includes voice, images, elements of a medical record, and commands to a surgical robot.[7]
> . . . the use of telecommunications technology, including satellite links, dedicated line connections, interactive television systems and Internet connections, to provide healthcare services to patients at some location separate from the provider.[8]
> . . . a composite term for health-related activities, services, and systems, carried out over a distance by means of information and communications technologies, for the purpose of global health promotion, disease control and healthcare, as well as education, management, and research for health.[9]

These definitions typify prevalent concepts of telemedicine at various times during the 1990s. They are useful as long as they are treated in appropriate historical context. But they are also static. None of the existing definitions captures the accelerating dynamism of the interface between communications, computers, information, and healthcare over the past few years. Consequently, with respect to the future, most previously published definitions of telemedicine are incomplete or oversimplified. They may show where telemedicine has been, but they fail to point in the direction where it is headed.

PROBLEMS WITH HISTORICAL DEFINITIONS

Typical definitions of telemedicine also fail to incorporate related changes that are taking place in other dimensions of healthcare delivery. For example, most attempts to explain the meaning of telemedicine are cast explicitly or implicitly in the context of a doctor-patient relationship. (Even the generic term *provider* is usually used as a synonym for doctor.) The physician-centric perspective misses one of the most significant long-term effects of the telemedicine revolution—the expanding clinical powers of nonphysician practitioners and of patients who will use telemedicine to access a knowledge base that has been controlled by medical doctors.[10] Hence, a future-focused definition must refer more broadly to caregivers or clinicians rather than just doctors. Definitions found in print in the 1990s will become irrelevant over the next few years because they assume a clinical hierarchy that will become progressively less important to the delivery of healthcare.

Telemedicine will be a great equalizer. It will expand dramatically the number of professionals who are independently qualified to make diagnostic and therapeutic decisions. Doctors will not be able to

---

TELEMEDICINE IS . . . ON MOUNT EVEREST

Nobody who has read *Into Thin Air,* Jon Krakauer's book about an ill-fated 1996 expedition to Everest, can forget the heartrending scene where a guide, about to die of exposure in a howling storm high on the mountain, reassures his pregnant wife in New Zealand by phone that he's okay. The sheer fact that they were able to communicate is a demonstration of the power and omnipresence of today's technology. But no amount of communications nor medical wizardry could have saved the lives of that brave climber and eleven of his comrades from the fatal combination of brutal weather and misjudgment that Krakauer so ably recounts. On the other hand, the more we learn about human physiology and performance under extreme conditions, the better prepared we may be to save lives in the future.

A team of vendors and academics—including AT&T, Logical Design Solutions, MIT, and Yale—pulled together the Everest Extreme Expedition (E3) to monitor climbers as they scale the world's tallest mountain. The system they designed collects data from physiologic sensors and digital video cameras carried by mountaineers and transmits it down to base camp clinic which is also equipped with a miniaturized intensive care unit, complete with a portable 3-D ultrasound. From base camp, data are

control telemedicine, nor will they be able to control other practitioners and patients who learn to use it. Many health professions will ultimately become masters of telemedicine as different independent practitioners learn to use this powerful tool within their own clinical models. Therefore, we refer throughout this book to the practitioner-patient relationship rather than the doctor-patient relationship because telemedicine will "level the playing field," giving both nonphysicians and patients access to medical knowledge that was once the protected domain of those who had graduated from medical school.

However, nonphysician health professionals such as nurses, dentists, pharmacists, and all varieties of therapists are not the only persons who will use telemedicine in expanding areas of clinical practice. Existing definitions are equally incomplete or misleading with respect to the future of healthcare when they fail to encompass consumer empowerment. Patients and their families are already joining the telemedicine revolution and dramatically reshaping medical services in the process. Consumers will become directly and deeply involved in their own healthcare. They will use telemedicine to change the practitioner-patient relationship in ways that few health professionals would have ever thought possible.

The twentieth century model of medical care—that is, the doctor defining the medical problem and deciding what to do about it—will be replaced by the twenty-first century model where many patients will make these decisions with assistance from a variety of practitioners

---

relayed to the INMARSAT satellite hovering over the Indian Ocean. INMARSAT rebroadcasts the signal to a land station in Malaysia which forwards it, via SATCOM Global network, to Santa Paula, California. The message is transmitted by ISDN links from California to experts at Yale and at Walter Reed Army Hospital.

Scientists at base camp (17,500 feet), and at Yale and Walter Reed (both near sea level) have been following climbers on the mountain, including four monitored volunteers who reached the summit (29,028 feet) in May 1998. You can visit the Everest Extreme Expedition at its Website, maintained by AT&T at www.att.com/everest/e3desc.html.

Because of the multiple vendors, many of whom have donated equipment and services to the project, the overall cost has not yet been determined. Likewise, much of the data has not been reviewed. In the final analysis, E3 may not have generated much scientific bang for the corporate buck. But then nobody ever tried to conquer Everest for reasons remotely related to cost-effectiveness. Certainly, this cooperative project is a fascinating demonstration of the ability of high-tech wizardry to collect and transmit medical data from anywhere on earth to anywhere else. To paraphrase Sir Edmund Hillary, maybe this technological mountain had to be climbed just because it's there.

(including doctors) and electronic decision-support tools. This empowerment of consumers is perhaps the most dramatic change that will be propelled by the revolution in healthcare communications, so it must be included in the definition of telemedicine. Consumer empowerment is, therefore, a major theme throughout this book.

Further, existing definitions and policy perspectives flowing from them tend to fall short of the mark because they do not address telemedicine's ability to overcome the longstanding barrier of time.[11] Definitions of telemedicine automatically encompass the barrier of distance because the Greek prefix, *teleo,* means far off or distant. However, the image conveyed by these definitions is problematic when it assumes that practitioners and the patient are required to participate in the encounter at the same time, albeit in different places (e.g., interactive television consultations).

Telemedicine creates a whole new realm of possibilities because it allows clinicians and patients to interact meaningfully at different times as well (e.g., "store and forward" exchange of clinical information). A word including the prefix *tempo* (meaning time) would actually be more appropriate in the context of our concern with looking to the future. However, we are probably too late to establish a word like *tempotelemedicine,* so we will be content with using the established word as long as readers remember that telemedicine breaks barriers of both distance and time.

Finally, the historical definitions do not address the economic dimension of telemedicine. At best, they assign no essential economic

---

TELEMEDICINE IS . . . RURAL–URBAN HEART LINK

Because it happens at the speed of light, electronic communications can make the distance between the sender and the receiver of a signal essentially irrelevant. A farsighted administration at Allen Memorial Hospital in Moab, Utah exploited this truism when it arranged to have data from patients in the hospital's intensive care unit brought up side-by-side with the data of patients at St. Mark's Hospital, 250 miles away in Salt Lake City. St. Mark's is a 306-bed tertiary care hospital, specializing in cardiac care. Allen Memorial boasts 38 beds, serving a community of approximately 9,000 and an enormous rural area that includes Arches National Park.

Once the link—dubbed SiteLink by Vital-Com, the commercial partner in this endeavor—was established in 1997, patients in Moab who required continuous monitoring of their cardiac status could take full advantage of the highly specialized intensive care nurses and subspecialist physicians at St. Mark's. Immediate access to such a high level of expertise is a rarity in a rural setting.

The system couples patient monitoring data with an interactive video connection between the staffs at both facilities. The fractional T-1 line linking the two

characteristics to telemedicine because they include no economic terminology. At worst, existing definitions imply that telemedicine is the next entry in a long list of expensive technologies that increase the costs of healthcare. The conceptual approach currently used by the Health Care Financing Administration (HCFA) is a case in point. Required by the Balanced Budget Act of 1997 to reimburse telemedicine-based specialty consultations for patients residing in underserved rural areas, HCFA has focused solely on the interactive video definition of telemedicine and has developed a restrictive payment formula based on the assumption that telemedicine will be financially ruinous unless tightly regulated.

HCFA's narrow, policy-focused definition diverts attention from the beneficial economic attributes of telemedicine. As will be demonstrated through this book's discussions and examples, telemedicine should be seen instead as a tool to eliminate waste and to improve outcomes—respectively defined as efficiency and effectiveness in the terminology of economic theory. The promise of telemedicine is better medical care at a lower cost. An ideal definition of telemedicine should reflect these microeconomic benefits.[12] (In an ideal world, HCFA would promulgate incentive-based policies that promote economically beneficial forms of telemedicine rather than punitive mechanisms that target interactive video, but we digress. . . .)

The emerging macroeconomic relationship between competition and telemedicine also merits explicit attention because it is central to the full meaning of telemedicine.[13] The early, simple concept of

---

sites also provides a dedicated phone and fax connection. But participants feel that the communication paraphernalia are merely infrastructure. The relationships and protocols that have been built between the two institutions and their staffs, facilitated by that high-tech infrastructure, are where the program's essence really lies.

Allen Memorial's CEO, Charles Davis, gives SiteLink much of the credit for saving his hospital which had been on the brink of closing because of low inpatient census. During the first five months of operation, high-level real-time monitoring was credited with reducing transfers from the intensive care unit by 82 percent, keeping an extra $80,000 at the local facility while saving an equal amount in patient transport costs. Furthermore, surgeons have been willing to perform higher risk surgeries locally, knowing that post-operative intensive care will be supported by some of the best experts in the state of Utah.

And nobody can place a value upon renewing the community's faith in Allen Memorial Hospital, one of Moab's cornerstone institutions. Telemedicine definitely helped to save it.

"medical care at a distance" makes no reference to the growing number of ways in which telemedicine will bring informed consumer choice, the essence of competition in economic theory, to the medical marketplace. Anyone who wants to know where telemedicine is leading us must understand how it will provide consumers with unprecedented options and the information to choose intelligently among them.

In other words, telemedicine will not only make existing systems more efficient by generating competition among them; it will drive development of whole new ways of organizing healthcare delivery. This proposition will perhaps be the hardest for traditionalists to grasp, so subsequent chapters will present considerable evidence in its support.

DEFINING TELEMEDICINE FOR THE FUTURE

To overcome the deficiencies of historical definitions in this rapidly evolving field, we have created a future-oriented definition to place telemedicine in proper perspective as one of the most powerful forces shaping a new, different, and better health system for the twenty-first century:

> Telemedicine is the combined use of telecommunications and computer technologies to improve the efficiency and effectiveness of healthcare services by liberating caregivers from traditional constraints of place and time and by empowering consumers to make informed choices in a competitive marketplace.

Numerous boxes are placed beneath the main text throughout the book to illustrate this definition by current example. These examples were specifically chosen to demonstrate the remarkable extent to which telemedicine has already permeated daily practice. The boxes should quickly expand the horizons of anyone who equates telemedicine with interactive television. Telemedicine is already much more than a closed-circuit, real-time video consultation between a rural patient and an urban specialist, and telemedicine will continue to expand rapidly in both depth and breadth.

Indeed, telemedicine will grow over the next few years to the point where ultimately it will be transparent to medical practice. The combined application of telecommunications and computer technologies will become so common that it will lose its current cachet as an area worthy of special concern. Telemedicine in its maturity will be an unnoticed context within which healthcare occurs.

This book describes how we will get from here to there, from today's widespread view of telemedicine as an enabling mechanism of rural health to tomorrow's general acceptance of telemedicine as a universal tool of the twenty-first century healthcare delivery system. Our comprehensive definition is essential to understanding the telemedicine revolution and participating intelligently in it because existing definitions have not encompassed its full scope.

Our approach is personalized throughout the book by the inclusion of biographical sketches of eleven living pioneers who have foreseen the power of telemedicine and dedicated extraordinary, career-defining efforts to pursuing their visions of its potential. We will undoubtedly come to regret our failure to feature other leaders who have done just as much, but the works of these eleven add a personal dimension to the definition of telemedicine within the confines of a book long enough to be informative but short enough to be interesting.

SEMANTIC VARIATIONS ON THE GENERAL THEME

Other terms, most notably *cybermedicine* and *telehealth,* have also been used by a few commentators during the 1990s. These designations are not necessarily intended to serve as synonyms for *telemedicine,* even though they generally employ the same technologies. Rather, these alternative terms are sometimes used to make a philosophical point, such as emphasizing a different perspective on the desired measure of the health system's final product. The means (i.e., the technologies) are the same, but the ends may be different.

For example, some prominent experts in the field have distinguished between telemedicine and telehealth on the basis of the group being served by the technology. Telemedicine is used to describe the realm of care-related applications that link patients and clinicians, while telehealth encompasses allied support functions:

> Telehealth includes clinical care but also encompasses the related areas of health professions education, consumer health education, public health, research, and administration. Telecommunications applications in this larger area include distance learning for degree and continuing education, both didactic lectures and clinical precepting; consumer health services, such as electronic support groups and consumer health information bulletin boards; administrative uses, including electronic billing and administrative conferencing; and telemedicine.[14]

In this formulation, telemedicine is the realm of technology that bridges gaps between clinicians and patients. Telehealth is the support system of electronic linkages between clinical care at a distance and the rest of the community.

Perhaps even more commonly, telehealth is used to emphasize the position that health—defined more than forty years ago by the World Health Organization (WHO) as a complete state of physical, mental, and social well-being, not just the absence of disease—ought to be the principal concern of public policy and resource allocation. It is used to highlight meaningful differences between the WHO's holistic concept of health and traditional medicine, the curatively oriented treatment of physical illness and injury. From this perspective, the technologies and related policy issues should be examined with respect to their contributions to the health of the community, not just the efficiency of the delivery system.

We are highly sympathetic to the long-run issues raised by this semantic nuance. Both authors have dedicated considerable effort over their professional lives to health promotion and disease prevention, healthy community programs, public health, professional education, and other activities based on the highly defensible position that keeping people healthy makes more economic and moral sense than waiting to treat them after they have become ill or injured.

However, to avoid being sidetracked by an idealistic debate over health versus medicine, we side with convention and use *telemedicine* throughout this book. Anyone offended by our editorial decision is missing the point. The revolution we describe in the following pages will change both medicine and health and blur the line between them.

TELEMEDICINE IS . . . WORKSITE WELLNESS

Many Americans with serious medical problems go to the Mayo Clinic, but how many Fortune 500 companies would turn to it for corporate wellness programs? Not many, you might think, because major corporations have employees all over the country, and Mayo has clinics in only three regions.

Think again, because telemedicine is creating new ways to promote health and prevent disease. It is allowing the Mayo Clinic to manage wellness programs throughout the world for Intel, Texas Instruments, Lucent Technologies, General Mills, and similar companies.

For most Americans, worksite wellness probably brings forth images of visits to the corporate health center for periodic risk assessments and follow-up meetings with a nurse to discuss modification of health behaviors. Now, with Mayo Clinic HealthQuest Online (800-430-9699; www.mhqprodinfo.org), face-to-face interaction is not the only viable option.

The new program uses a computerized "Personal Health Scorecard" to help employees identify areas for self-improvement, provides different types of on-line information to promote health, and monitors progress toward desired goals. Individualized "Disease Management Planners" are also a part of the interactive network so that workers—including those with chronic conditions—can assume more responsibility for taking care of themselves.

Telemedicine will affect all areas of human health, from the broadest perspectives of community health to the narrowest subspecialties of allopathic medicine, from twentieth century Western medicine to healing traditions from other times and places. It will also change health professions education, medical care organization, and health administration. Quibbling over narrow definitions is a waste of time because the joint impact of computers and telecommunications will be experienced in all areas—regardless of the name assigned to any particular area of special interest.

TELEMEDICINE AND MEDICAL INFORMATICS

Another term, *telematics,* also appears occasionally in materials that address the technological transformation of medicine. It is obviously a compound word derived from telemedicine and informatics. Although the two subjects are closely related and often overlapping, they are not identical. A brief overview of medical informatics reveals not only the similarities and the differences, but also the many ways in which telemedicine and informatics will increasingly complement each other.

HealthQuest allows companies to customize the site to address internal health promotion efforts or special problems—such as a flu outbreak affecting workers in one office or factory—and promptly disseminate information about preventive measures. The site also includes links to self-care information, and participating companies can add the capability for workers to talk to a nurse whenever they feel the need for something more than a computer connection.

Other significant features of telemedical corporate wellness include twenty-four-hour-a-day availability and standardization of on-line services. Regardless of shift or location, any employee can conveniently access the full range of available information. In addition, computer-based systems are being used to conduct ongoing cross-sectional studies, to identify significant relationships between health behaviors and employee characteristics across the company to manage targeted interventions, and to monitor the interventions. This new set of capabilities can produce programmatic changes faster and cheaper than traditional approaches to wellness.

Of course, networked computers can't do aerobic exercises or prepare more healthful meals, but now they can help employees explore more options and make better choices. Many other progressive healthcare organizations will undoubtedly join the Mayo Clinic in developing a whole new range of on-line services that empower individuals to improve health on their own terms.

Informatics is the applied science of collecting, storing, and retrieving data to support informed decision-making.[15] It has been developed as a specialized field in most major industries, including healthcare. Informatics enables the use of modern information sciences and related technologies to optimize a wide range of production and marketing activities. It transforms data from simple records of what happened in the past into rich information about possibilities for the future—identifying everything from better ways to combine inputs to new systems that improve the health of target populations.

The theories behind informatics (e.g., the content of many modern economics and business courses) have been around for decades in the works of well-known writers like Juran, Deming, Arrow, and Drucker. However, the transformation from graduate-level academic principles into widespread business practices required the more recent arrival of three technologies: computers, networks, and digitization.

- *Computers:* Modern computer systems provide us with unprecedented power to analyze data and create information. In comparison to the inaccessible and expensive mainframes that filled large rooms until the mid-1980s, today's personal computers (desktops, laptops, and palmtops) make data available to virtually everyone involved in production and sales. Best of all, the costs of computing have fallen dramatically. The computer industry keeps delivering products that are smaller, faster, and cheaper. Healthcare may be behind other industries in developing the computer power to match its abundant data, but conditions are ripe for fast growth.

- *Networks:* The rapid development of digital switches and software that create networks by linking computers is just as important to the intertwined futures of medical informatics and telemedicine. Computers can now "talk" to each other in ways that were unimaginable less than a decade ago.[16] The decline of the floppy disk drive (from built-in component to optional peripheral in less than two years!) and the corresponding rise of the modem are sure signs of the fundamental importance of networks.

- *Digitization:* The technology to transform all healthcare data into a common form, expressed as combinations of 0 and 1 (the digits of the binary number system), is the third advance that opens informatics and telemedicine to revolutionary possibilities. Computers have stored and processed numbers

and letters in binary files for approximately fifty years, but
images and sounds—very important elements in the total
practice of medicine—have been stored almost exclusively (if
they were stored at all) on acetate film, paper, or recording
tape until the 1990s. Now, at the end of the twentieth century,
technology exists to reduce the visual and aural elements of
human health to the same digital formats used for text and
data files since the advent of computers. A practitioner's sense
of touch can be encoded, stored, and recreated digitally
through haptic feedback devices. Finally, clinicians and
researchers can explore all medical information in one format,
at the same time, and in one convenient location (e.g., at a
single work station).

Medical informatics and telemedicine are both advanced dramatically by these three technological developments, but they are still
likely to remain separate domains for the foreseeable future. Medical
informatics will improve the efficiency and effectiveness of processes
that produce medical services. Telemedicine will change the product
and transform relationships that define the healthcare industry. A
medical services provider with state-of-the-art capabilities in medical
informatics will not necessarily be involved in telemedicine and vice
versa.

The relationship between medical informatics and telemedicine
will become increasingly synergistic. Progressive healthcare organizations will be expanding their capabilities in both of these areas.
Telematics will continue to be the name for the overlapping interface
between them but will not be a synonym for either.

TELEMEDICINE IN EVOLVING PRACTICE

As noted in the foregoing comparison with medical informatics,
telemedicine is more than a new tool to improve the production of existing goods and services. Telemedicine is enabling the creation of a
whole new concept of healthcare in its rapid translation from theory
into practice. The ultimate promise of telemedicine is to allow us to
find new ways to take care of our physical, mental, and social needs.
That it will allow us to do some old things more efficiently along the
way must not obscure the fact that it is the engine of remarkable
change. Healthcare will never be the same after telemedicine has matured over the next few years. The whole realm of human health will
be radically different.

The telemedicine revolution is not happening in a social or economic vacuum. It is closely linked to—although lagging behind, in some significant cases—comparable upheavals in banking, entertainment, education, shopping, and other activities of everyday life in the developed, post-industrial world. In the insightful words of Michael Vlahos, telemedicine is part of a larger transformation in time and space:

> In short, our new tools are building a new place and we are moving there. The technologies of the "Information Revolution" are not simply altering our world at the margins by improving how we communicate and share data between old places, but they are creating a new world that is an actual place to which people are migrating.[17]

By extension, telemedicine is already and will continue to be an international phenomenon. Some notable developments are occurring outside the United States, available for adoption here when regulatory barriers are lowered or when foreign entrepreneurs decide to tackle our markets. On the other hand, American hardware and software are

TELEMEDICINE IS . . . DISTANCE TEACHING

Since 1995 the High Plains Rural Health Network (HPRHN) has been installing the infrastructure—video hardware, T-1 lines, protocols, and support—for an ambitious video system that links most of the northeast quadrant of Colorado and neighboring bits of Kansas, Nebraska, and Wyoming with tertiary hospitals along the urban front range corridor of Colorado. North Colorado Family Medicine, the family practice residency training program in Greeley, Colorado, has been one of the heaviest users of the network. Interactive video has become a crucial strategy employed to support the residency's mission to train rural family doctors.

Wray lies 148 miles from Greeley, on the far eastern edge of Colorado. With a population of approximately 2,000 residents, Wray is the smallest town in the United States with a full-time graduate medical training program. Rural training track residents spend their first year in Greeley and their last two years in Wray, where they get the sort of real small town practice experience that could only be obtained in a real small town.

Getting plenty of exposure to patients with a wide range of medical needs is no problem in the thriving Wray practice. On the other hand, supporting the resident with the lectures and oversight that are an integral part of the home program in Greeley has been a challenge. This is where interactive video fits in.

Beginning in 1996, the rural training track residents have "attended" Wednesday afternoon lectures in Greeley without leaving Wray via a video link provided by HPRHN. As a bonus, the presentations have been beamed from the residency conference room to the resident call room in the hospital across the street, allowing on-call residents who must remain in-house to participate. According to Dr. Dan Fahrenholz, director of the Rural Training Track, residents at all three sites participate equally and unselfconsciously.

probably the most common elements in telemedical applications throughout the world. Notwithstanding protectionist trade barriers erected to shelter national or regional economic entities, we can expect the telemedicine revolution to make many of its dramatic changes without respect to international borders. Computers don't have nationalities, nor do the telecommunications networks that already tie the world together.

Telemedicine at home and abroad will evolve so quickly and so extensively over the next few years that any effort to contain it misses the point of the revolution. As has been noted by many leading commentators on the information age, computers and networks are creating many discontinuities. The time warp between those who develop the new technologies and those who try to regulate them is particularly problematic. Bureaucrats simply cannot keep up with computer engineers, software developers, and system designers (a problem addressed in later chapters).

When not being used for lectures, the video unit is rolled down to the room in the residency's clinic where faculty are available to teach residents in the process of seeing patients. Rural Training Track residents in Wray have the same access to these teachers as the Greeley residents (assuming that somebody has remembered to move the unit into the precepting room and turn it on, which, unfortunately, still doesn't happen all the time—another example of the prime importance of convenience and simplicity to any information system.)

Trainees in Wray use the system mostly to do "talking head" questions and answers with faculty in Greeley. Occasionally they have employed the system to demonstrate a patient's physical finding, such as a rash. An otoscope/ophthalmoscope attachment allows preceptors in Greeley to see the eardrums and retinas of patients in Wray—displayed on a full size video monitor and "frozen" as electronic "slides"—with greater clarity than they can see on patients at the home clinic. When not consulting in real-time, remote trainees have captured images of skin lesions, ears, and eyes, stored them, and forwarded them to Greeley for later discussion with faculty. A headband-mounted camera that will allow remote faculty to "be" with the resident and patient in the exam room is in the works.

In 1998, the Residency Review Commission for Family Medicine gave the Rural Training Track Program full accreditation. Video conferencing and precepting figured critically in the application and approval. The accrediting body, understandably a little timid about fully embracing the concept of virtual teachers, did not comment in its report on the use of video technology. But the accreditors seemed satisfied that the medical residents in Wray were getting the support and supervision they needed to enable them to become excellent family doctors. Residents and faculty wholeheartedly agree.

Healthcare is no exception to this general rule, so readers who want or need to understand the future of telemedicine must not become distracted by bureaucratic determinations of what is permissible in the short-run. The future of healthcare lies in what telemedicine makes possible now and in the future. The marriage of computers and telecommunications is spawning an exciting increase in the realm of possibilities on all sides of the market. This book is intended not only to justify the enthusiasm of visionary reformers, but to challenge the thinking of those who would regulate the development of telemedicine for fear of losing control.

Why a book?

From our point of view as authors tackling such a dynamic topic, the task of writing this book is somewhat like the conundrum faced by anyone considering the purchase of a computer. If the prospective buyer waits just a little bit longer before making the purchase, more features will be available for less money. On the other hand, the result of continued waiting for the next advancement or discount is never owning a computer. The price one pays to play in today's high-tech world is the expectation—nay, the certainty—that the machine bought today will be replaced by something better and cheaper within a few weeks following the date of purchase.

We know that if we wait just a little longer to write this book, new applications of telemedicine are certain to emerge. These noteworthy advancements will make some sections of this book seem dated within weeks of its publication. Ironically, this predictable obsolescence is an important part of our basic message. Telemedicine will expand in scope and revolutionize healthcare faster than it possibly can be followed in a book. Traditional print media operate at a slower speed than the electronic technologies that are replacing them.

Why, then, aren't we writing an electronic "book?" The answer to this question illustrates paradoxes that attach almost universally to times of sudden and radical change. The French, a people experienced in revolutions, have an expression that puts the situation in useful perspective: *Le plus ça change, le plus c'est la même chose.* ("The more things change, the more they stay the same.") The tools of the *ancien régime* are used to overthrow it, but they never totally disappear. In analogous scientific terms, such inconsistencies are the stuff of progress.[18] Our book may help pave the way for new, nonprint types of publications in the future because it describes how things can and will be different.

For the time being, most of the medical care leaders and interested "outsiders" who need to understand telemedicine are still dependent on books. They are not yet fluent in the use of the electronic media that will rapidly transform the foundations of human health. If we were to distribute this book in an electronic format, we would be preaching to a small (but growing) choir of on-line clinicians and administrators who already know what we are talking about. In other words, an electronic book would be seen by those who don't need it—bypassing the much larger group of not-yet-wired individuals who will benefit from its message.

The rapid development of telecomputing has given rise to a new definition of an old term, *convergence*. The ongoing merger of the television set and the computer terminal is a good example of convergence technology, as is the migration of fax machine, photocopier, and document scanner into a single unit.[19] We have written this book with an analogous goal in mind. Departing from the linear model of traditional books, we have attempted to translate into print some of the nonlinear devices employed in electronic media such as Web pages. This book's boxes, creative layouts, pioneer profiles, glossary, and annotated references are consistent with the print publishing industry's movement in the direction of its own special version of user-friendly convergence.

We certainly cannot yet claim that our medium is the message, but we have tried to bridge the gap with a view to the electronic future wherever possible. And even if you were reading this text on-line or listening to it over the Internet as an audio file while watching linked images on a 3-D video headset, we as authors would not want the message to be obscured by the technology. Writing anything about today's technology-driven trends is extraordinarily difficult because historical epochs may literally be measured in weeks or months. Thanks to independent advances in telecommunications and computing, things are about to get crazy in the world of healthcare.

Overview of the book

The next step in our inquiry into the past, present, and future of telemedicine is a hypothetical look back at healthcare over the next two decades from the perspective of 2020. Using the device of a letter from a physician to her son who is contemplating a career in medicine, Chapter 2 presents a "big picture" view of changes that are likely to be wrought by telemedicine, with a special emphasis on some of the underlying human issues.

Since this book is about a revolution, Chapter 3 explores the general concept of dramatic technological change and examines specific links between the Industrial Revolution era that we are leaving and the Information Revolution that we are now entering. It also presents the broad social and political context within which healthcare will be transformed over the next few years. Chapter 4 then links the Seventh Revolution, telemedicine, with the six previous scientific and technological advances that have redefined medical practice and healthcare in the modern era.

Chapter 5 is the core of the book, tying together the "Telemedicine is. . ." boxes that appear throughout these pages. It provides a detailed analysis of telemedicine's likely impact on everything from healthcare information and medical records to research, health insurance, and the reorganization of the delivery system. This chapter also elaborates one of the book's most important points, the transformational impact of empowered consumers and resulting shifts in the balance of power between professionals who produce healthcare and customers who buy it.

Chapter 6 focuses on the technological foundations of telemedicine. It explains the workings of hardware, software, and other components of computer systems that are being developed for clinical applications, and it explores the basic communications equipment and networks that give telemedicine its unprecedented power to liberate healthcare from long-standing barriers of time and place. Chapter 6 concludes with practical discussion of seven specific keys to success for readers who will be responsible for planning and implementing telemedicine projects. Chapter 7 then explores key economic and sociopolitical issues raised by the Seventh Revolution, including the future of payment for telemedicine and several dimensions of consumer protection. This chapter concludes with an actual example of guidelines being used to promote the quality of telemedical services.

Chapter 8 is an annotated list of references and resources that will be particularly helpful to anyone who wants to learn more about telemedicine and keep up with rapid developments in the field. Chapter 9 concludes the book with an extensive glossary of key terms and their meanings so that readers will be able to participate meaningfully in discussions of telemedicine.

NOTES

1. Murphy, RL, TB Fitzpatrick, HA Hayes, et al. "Accuracy of dermatologic diagnosis by television," *Archives of Dermatology* 105(6):833–835 (1972).

2. Dr. Jane Preston, founding president of the American Telemedicine Association, described these three earlier programs in her book, *The Telemedicine Handbook: Improving Health Care with Interactive Video* (Austin, Tex.: Telemedical Interactive Consultative Services, Inc., 1993), 4–6. Her book provides references to the original published descriptions of these early projects.

3. Ibid., 1.

4. Lindbergh, Donald (Director, National Library of Medicine) in testimony to the U.S. House of Representatives, Committee on Science, Space, and Technology, Subcommittee on Oversight and Investigations, May 2, 1994.

5. Grigsby, J, RE Schlenker, MM Kaehny, PW Shaugnessy, EJ Sandberg. "Analytic Framework for Evaluation of Telemedicine," *Telemedicine Journal* 1:31–39 (1995).

6. U.S. Department of Commerce, National Telecommunications and Information Administration, *A Nation of Opportunity: Realizing the Promise of the Information Superhighway.* U.S. Government Printing Office, 1996.

7. Coiera, E. *Guide to Medical Informatics, the Internet, and Telemedicine* (New York: Chapman and Hall Medical, 1997) as quoted in *Journal of the American Medical Association* 280(15): 1367 (October 21, 1998).

8. *A Glossary of Health Care Terms,* 3 ed. (Boston, Mass: Goulston & Storrs, 1997).

9. World Health Organization, "A Health Telmatics Policy." Report of the WHO Group Consultation on Health Telematics, Geneva, (December 11–16, 1997), 1.

10. For a detailed analysis of the expanding independence of nonphysician clinicians, see Jeffrey C. Bauer, *Not What the Doctor Ordered: How to End the Medical Monopoly in Pursuit of Managed Care* (New York: McGraw-Hill, 1998).

11. A few recent review articles are beginning to give proper recognition to the time dimension. For example, see JC Kvedar, E Menn, and KR Loughlin. "Telemedicine: Present Applications and Future Prospects," *Urologic Clinics of North America* 25(1):137–149 (February 1998). Their analysis is based from the very beginning on a time and place-independent view of information technology. (However, it is entirely focused on a physician-centered view of healthcare delivery.)

12. Microeconomics is the study of production (supply) and consumption (demand). On the supply side of the market,

production theory addresses key issues like finding the least-expensive combinations of inputs and optimizing returns on investments in capital investments. Demand-side analysis seeks to explain consumers' behavior with respect to price, income, and variables that reflect satisfaction and expectations. Production and consumption theories come together in the "law of supply and demand," a general model which explains how price and quantity are set in markets for individual goods and services. Elimination of waste is a key measure of success in microeconomic analysis.

13. Macroeconomics addresses the "big picture," focusing on issues like the sum total of all final microeconomic activity (gross domestic product, or GDP) and government actions to influence microeconomic decisions (e.g., monetary policy via the Treasury and Federal Reserve System, fiscal policy implemented through government spending, and tax policy). Macroeconomics is also concerned with a nation's overall economic welfare, so it encompasses antitrust policy and related government powers to regulate producer actions that restrict consumer choice.

14. Puskin, DS, CL Mintzer, and CJ Wasem "Telemedicine: Building Rural Systems for Today and Tomorrow" in PF Brennan, SJ Schneider, and E Tornquist. *Information Networks for Community Health* (New York: Springer-Verlag, 1997), 275–276. This source draws its definitional differences between telemedicine and telehealth in the context of the *televillage,* a useful metaphor that draws attention to even broader linkages between healthcare and the rest of the community.

15. Bauer, JC, WT Brown, and P Zimnik. "Wave of informatics will transform profession," *Dental Economics* (August, 1998), 113.

16. For a fascinating study of the people and processes that created network computing, see K Hafner and M Lyon, *Where Wizards Stay Up Late: The Origins of the Internet* (New York: Simon & Schuster, 1996).

17. Michael Vlahos. "Entering the Infosphere," *Journal of International Affairs* 51(2):501 (Spring 1998).

18. Readers who care to pursue the fascinating implications of this tangential point will likely enjoy Douglas Hofstadter's classic work, *Godel, Escher, Bach: An Eternal Golden Braid* (New York: Basic Books, 1979).

19. The concept of convergence is extending even into unexpected realms. For example, Michel Lemieux and Victor Pilon are in the

process of developing a new form of stage entertainment that merges traditional theater and the same telecomputing technologies that enable telemedicine. Their 1999 play, *Orféo,* has gained considerable attention in both the United States and Canada because it simultaneously presents live actors and virtual actors (i.e., remote in time and place) on the stage. The multidimensional experience of this Lemieux-Pilon production shows that healthcare is not the only part of our lives being revolutionized by new technologies. Art and science are both affected.

2 CHAPTER

A Letter from the Future (2020 Hindsight)

Northeast Colorado Family Health Center
Brush, Colorado 80723
March 27, 2020

Dear Son,

You will surely wonder why I am communicating on your twenty-first birthday in the old-fashioned way, text-only E-mail, and why I have chosen to dust off my old computer keyboard and type this greeting when I could have dictated it to my wrist-top computerphone in about one-tenth the time. Well, your old mom hasn't gone completely crazy. A multimedia version is on its way to your home entertainment center for you to view this evening, but I do want to make a point about the future as you start this special day.

I remember getting a twenty-first birthday letter written on my father's typewriter—a big, clunky thing he used until he retired. (He had an employee called a secretary who then retyped all his drafts, if you can believe it!) When he struck a key, a molded piece of metal struck an inked ribbon and created the corresponding letter or number on a sheet of paper wrapped around a spool that had to be advanced mechanically each time a line was completed. Mistakes had to be covered with a paper-colored paint called correction fluid.

Invented at the end of the nineteenth century and surviving as state-of-the-art technology for nearly one hundred years, the typewriter was a great leap forward in the efficiency and legibility of personal communications (in comparison with writing by hand). Consequently, I donated Dad's typewriter to the Museum of Physical Reality in Aspen. You can go touch this relic on your next ski vacation. You'll be surprised at the feel of its keyboard and the loud noise it makes.

When I was at the university, we wrote papers by banging away on the keyboard of a personal computer. They literally were papers because the last step was to print our work on paper and give it to the teacher. Programs called word processors allowed us to write and edit on a screen, eliminating the need for correction fluid. Back in the typewriter age, some people made a living by typing papers for students and charging by the page. With the arrival of word processors, some critics feared that easy editing would lead to shallow thought because writers would not have to worry about the inconveniences of mechanical correction. Then again, when the typewriter was introduced, people who wrote by hand complained of the machine's distracting clatter and speed.

I still love to write at a keyboard. You may think that writing one letter at a time is old-fashioned, but I compare it somewhat to your decision to learn to play a real wooden cello rather than learning to program the same musical sounds with a digital music system. I love my turn-of-the-century keyboard and outdated word processing software as much as you love your old wooden cello. Just as writers used to say they could think better with pen in hand, I can think better with this familiar keyboard at my fingertips.

And think I must as you contemplate following in my footsteps and those of my father before me. I really want to say the right things to you before you graduate from college and take your first steps toward a career in medicine. I've been there for a lot of your first steps, including your real ones when you were a baby.

My father was not there for my first steps. He was a busy doctor in what he thought was the "golden age" of medicine, the 1950s through the 1980s. To be the good doctor that he was, he had to be physically present with his patients almost all the time—at the bedside, in the office, in the operating room. When he wasn't with his patients, he was constantly distracted by the ringing of the proverbial "phone on the wall." (Telephones used to be permanently wired into wall-mounted boxes.) As a child, I came to hate the sound of a ringing telephone because, more often than not, it meant Daddy had to leave. But it defined the way medicine was practiced in the second half of the twentieth century.

I remember having this career discussion with my father many years ago, just as I'm having it now with you. "What does it mean to be a doctor," I asked? I'll never forget his answer. "To be a doctor is, above all, to have the privilege of entering your patients' lives. It is the most human thing you can do, and one of the most noble, to use all of your learning, skills, and intuition to help alleviate suffering. No matter how much we know, there will always be magic in the relationship between doctor and patient." I cannot say it any better than he did.

Fortunately for me and for you, I have not had to repeat my father's personal sacrifices in striving to meet such very high expectations for a successful career in medicine. The telemedicine revolution has been a true blessing to me. You may not see it as a revolution, taking for granted all the things you use that are made "smart" by the computer chips embedded in them.

I even noticed that your new mountain bike's shocks and gears adjust automatically to the terrain. This reminds me of the bicycle store near the small northeastern Colorado town where I grew up. Its repair shop had a number of tools that were all powered by one electric motor. The owner had to be a mechanic just to run the machine that did all the bicycle work. He certainly couldn't just drop in a new chip to correct a problem. Fixing things required manual skill and, more often than not, spare parts.

Today's digital world sure is different! When I was

training in the 1990s, about five years before you were born and back when dinosaurs roamed the earth (as you used to kid me when you were in grade school), personal computers were big boxes that sat on our desks. We had to learn how to connect them to "peripherals" with clunky cables and how to install our own software from "disks." To use each advance in hardware and software, we had to climb what we called a "learning curve." New programs required us to learn new commands to be typed into the computers on our desks.

As archaic as this process may seem to you, it was still a big improvement over the state of computers that existed when I was a child. The original computers cost millions of dollars, filled large rooms, needed their own air-conditioning systems, and received their instructions from paper cards. Regular citizens never even got close to these machines. Graduate students of that era carried cardboard boxes full of punch cards to store their data and enter them into the computer. By the time I entered college, we had happily progressed to floppy disks, little plastic contraptions that contained our programs and data files. Some of us even had our own "personal" computers.

Data entry was a persistent problem. We could almost count on it not working right the first time. Software vendors established "customer support lines," phone numbers we called for troubleshooting help where—if we were lucky—we wouldn't have to wait more than half an hour to talk to somebody. If we were really lucky, the person was actually able to solve our problem. We also had to fight the operating system to get devices to "talk" to each other every time we changed a printer, monitor, input device, or any other part of the computer.

Then along came the Internet, the precursor of the Universal Wide-Band ComNet that you use today. Its protocols allowed dispersed computers to communicate over telephone lines. But getting two distant computers to talk to each other initially was more challenging than getting a computer to work with its printer. Lots of time was spent in troubleshooting.

The situation was especially rough for doctors in rural practice when I finished my residency and started my practice in Brush. We had limited access to the experts who could make systems run. We also didn't have much bandwidth, something your generation takes for granted. Most communication was done over "twisted pairs," the copper wires that connected telephones for most of the twentieth century. A pair of wires handled data at a very limited rate, so engineers had to learn to compress data at one end of the pipeline and decompress it at the other end. Eight bundled pairs, called a T1 line, could transmit sound and jerky, poor quality video at a high price. This red herring prevented many analysts from foreseeing the truly revolutionary implications of telemedicine.

Fiberoptic cable was becoming more common in the years just before you were born. By the time you entered kindergarten, wireless service with wide "data pipes" allowed us rural folk to transmit not only high quality images but also information formatted for multimedia and virtual reality. Until that time, however, the life of a small town doctor could be pretty difficult.

Imagine what practice was like for me in the days before telemedicine became the ubiquitous and transparent tool that it is today. For example, I frequently faced tense situations in the middle of the night with a patient who had been injured in a car wreck. I had to rely on what I had learned in a two-day trauma course to interpret the victim's neck X ray. I did not have the luxury of time to send the film to a radiologist. That's right, *film* . . . the image wasn't even digital! If I missed a fracture—an easy thing to do in a structure as complicated as a three-dimensional neck projected onto two-dimensional film—the patient ran the risk of being paralyzed. And I ran the risk of a guilty conscience and a ruined reputation.

Given such circumstances, getting doctors to practice in rural areas was a problem throughout the last three decades of the twentieth century. We all trained in big urban medical centers, like nothing you'll ever see if you decide to go to medical school. We were surrounded by subspecialists and machines of every sort. If we encountered an unfamiliar problem in medical school or residency training, we could always order the latest test and count on the right specialist showing up at the hospital when we called him. (Most of our teachers were men at that time.)

Those of us who decided to practice in the boondocks were not entirely on our own. Telephone contact with urban-based specialists helped overcome some problems, albeit awkwardly in many instances. The specialists could answer a lot of questions and talk us through some pretty rough situations. I once delivered a breech baby with the nurse holding the telephone receiver to my ear while an obstetrician in Denver gave me step-by-step instructions for accomplishing this difficult and dangerous maneuver.

Starting a year or two before you were born, the Internet gave rural practitioners the opportunity to use E-mail to communicate about less urgent issues. I could send a question to a specialist and then review the answer at my leisure. I could also attach a digital picture file to the E-mail message. At first, the quality of the photos was not always sufficient for definitive diagnosis, and the size of the files meant slow transmission. However, digital photography quickly got cheaper, better, and faster. Grandma and Grandpa were absolutely amazed at the quality of the baby photo I E-mailed to them when you were less than one hour old!

The pace of technological progress in the acquisition and transfer of digital images took off from there at a stunning rate. By the time you took your first steps just ten months later, I E-mailed to my parents a thirty second video clip of the event that very same day! (The length of the clip was not limited by the technology. Like the Wright brothers on their first flight, you didn't stay up very long.) I remember that we doctors initially had trouble keeping up with the fast-paced development of our abilities to use digital images to improve medical records, clinical consults, and patient education. The rate of technological progress at the turn-of-the-century was truly breathtaking; it virtually (pardon the pun) caught us by surprise.

The electronic revolution in medical information and communications came none too soon for us stubbornly proud rural doctors. Of course, we already had our libraries of books, hopefully with editions that were not too many years out of date. In the mid-1990s many of us started to acquire CD-ROMs, little silvery disks that contained a whole lot more data than floppy disks. Subscription services supplied us with new disks as often as every few months, making the information we used that much fresher.

But, since a computer was not yet part of every medical device (or bicycle), we had to go back to our office and "fire-up" our personal computer in order to get the information we needed from the CD-ROMs. We might even search the National Library of Medicine database, accessing it over the Internet with our personal computers in our "spare time." (Today's capability to get all information through the computer phones we wear on our belts is one of the most significant advances in medical technology.)

I am talking only about medical information, not patient information. Most medical records were still paper documents when you were a toddler at the beginning of the millennium, meaning we doctors had to find an actual chart—a sheaf of collated papers—in order to learn about our patients. In my small practice, the staff spent hours every day tracking down information which had not arrived from the laboratory, getting reports from consulting physicians, arranging schedules with the hospital, handling financial details with insurance companies, etc. Electronic medical records with complete and up-to-date information on every patient were not universally available until about the time you entered grade school.

What changes I've seen since the healthcare industry discovered computers and telecommunications! Once I got good at encoding all patient data in an electronic format, I could transmit any part of the record at the speed of light to any site where it was needed. Then I started embedding automatic reminders and routines in the record, to be sure that patients were getting their immunizations, that their drugs did not have adverse interactions, and that lab tests were ordered when they were needed (even when I got distracted by other duties, such as attending your grade school programs).

I must admit that we physicians who trained in the twentieth century were dragged, kicking and screaming, into the electronic age. We needed several years to overcome long-standing traditions like handwritten records and blind faith in our ability to remember everything. Other information-intensive industries, like banking and aviation, were several decades ahead of medicine in recognizing the value of the digital revolution.

When I went to medical school, we were still expected to memorize endless tangles of biochemical pathways and infinitely dividing courses of arteries, veins, and nerves. I'd forgotten most of it before I completed my residency

in the mid-1990s. If you decide to make yourself the third
generation of our family to enter medicine, you will be
spared most of this pain. Your professors will teach from
the twenty-first century premise that what you really need
to know is how to find out what you need to know. And finding
out what you need to know is so much easier than it used
to be. (Be grateful that you will never need to pretend
that you already know it all simply because you are a
doctor.)

What can you expect at the health sciences center where
you will begin your training, if you decide to become a
doctor? First, alongside classmates from the other schools
of advanced professional practice like pharmacy, nursing,
dentistry, and psychology, you will learn the general theory
of how the human body works. As you refine your understanding
of deviations from desirable function and specialize in the
medical model, you will learn how to ask diagnostic questions and where to get the best information to answer them.
Computer networks will give you access to a realm of knowledge that was not available when my generation was in medical school.

Remember that your patients will also have access to
most, if not all, of the same information. Your job will be
to help them make informed decisions based on their own
values and individual potential for physical, mental, social, and spiritual well-being. Even at the end of the twentieth century, patient empowerment basically meant the patient's right to choose a doctor. We physicians actually
believed that patients did not and could not understand
health, that they were totally dependent on us. We all grew
up in an era when "doctor knows best" and "just what the
doctor ordered" were common phrases of everyday speech. Back
when you were born in 1999, we couldn't begin to imagine how
quickly telemedicine would create the different type of empowered patient served by health practitioners over the past
ten to fifteen years.

The decision-making process embedded in the tools you
and your patients will use to analyze patient data—we used
to call it artificial intelligence—will lead to the correct diagnosis and treatment recommendations most of the
time. In fact, your patients' own current entries into
their virtual medical records, coupled with their up-to-

date health data profiles, will regularly produce correct answers without your intervention. Today's virtual systems arguably make better diagnostic and therapeutic decisions than I did in my first decade of practice in the 1990s. Faster and cheaper, too.

So, why do we even need doctors and other advanced-practice health professionals? Because well-trained humans can still do some things better than a machine can. Because talented individuals like you are filled with potential for empathy and understanding. Because medical training has finally focused on enhancing the traits that make you human, those things that will make you a healer.

Medical education in my day was characterized by long hours, sleep deprivation, insecurity, and public put-downs by superiors. We left twentieth century medical school less human and less able to heal others than when we started. I've spent my whole career unlearning some of the toxic lessons of medical training. Because we now have the luxury of instant access to the data we need—without the constraints that tied your grandfather and me to the clinic, the hospital, and the appointment book—authority and hierarchy count for a whole lot less than they did when I learned to do something simply because my instructors said it was the thing to do.

Now, two decades into the twenty-first century, many non-physicians seem to have as much credibility as the august medical school professors of my day. My doctor's-eye view of the traditional hierarchy changed dramatically when I brought the acupuncturist into my practice around 2005. I still don't understand much about what he does or why he does it, and I don't know if I'll ever be able to distinguish a "slippery" pulse from a "wiry" one. But my comprehensive practice data profile shows that he has cured a number of patients I might not have been able to help at all with my medical knowledge. Acupuncture was exotic, even distrusted, back then. Today, thanks to information technology, it is just another of the many modalities we use in my practice.

Thinking about this change reminds me of a night around Thanksgiving in 1998 when I couldn't sleep because you were kicking me nonstop *in utero*. I stayed awake for hours reading an unprecedented issue of the *Journal of the*

American Medical Association, one containing nothing but studies of alternative therapies that were opposed by traditional medicine. *JAMA's* reports of successful treatments involving Chinese moxibustion, vitamin therapy, and herbal remedies were absolutely shocking to my scientifically trained sensibilities. I have kept that issue of *JAMA* because I think it played a major role in giving legitimacy to integrative medicine in its infancy. Who knows? Maybe some of my new thoughts that night were transferred to you through the umbilical cord, adding a mystical explanation for your lifelong interest in becoming a doctor.

Your experience with medical training would surely be quite different from mine. I nevertheless worry about you being a minority—not because of your darker skin (which actually puts you in the majority now), but because so few males are becoming doctors these days. Medicine has become much more of a women's profession at the same time it has been demystified by automation and communications technology. I wonder how you young men might be traumatized by reverse sexism. (This would be a transgenerational case of "what goes around, comes around" because my father and his comrades certainly traumatized the few women in their class.) I don't suppose it's politically correct for a woman of mixed race to say this, but I remain concerned about keeping a balance between males and females in medicine. We still haven't learned enough about dealing with the social dimensions of technology.

Still, given the way telemedicine has revolutionized and improved healthcare since I entered practice, I think medical training is worth the trouble. I've had a wonderful career, especially in the last ten years. I have all the benefits of living in the same rural area where I grew up and where my father practiced. But, thanks to technology, I have immediate access to medical resources that my father never dreamed of having. The laboratory work and imaging we do here are every bit as sophisticated as what they do at the urban medical centers. The interpretations are just as fast and just as good, too. And I don't need a computer network specialist to help me get them. The system is 100% user-friendly.

All of us in my practice use the same clinical protocols, constantly updated on the basis of ongoing patient experience and tailored to my practice population. After all, I would be wasting everyone's time if I told my rancher patients with artery disease to quit eating beef, so I program their home monitoring services to help them regulate their blood chemistry in other ways. The ability to interact with patients through their individualized databases has really helped cut costs and improve quality.

And how I love my international practice. As you know, I've been studying tropical diseases as a hobby for years. I'm now an active member of the multidisciplinary team that is addressing the latest malaria epidemic in northern Brazil. I can do my consultations from home or from the office—thanks to real-time access to the sights, sounds, feel, and even smells of the distant people I am treating. Virtual reality still isn't quite the same as being there, but it is getting awfully close. Although I have never visited the Amazon clinic where I am volunteering my time, I know the clinical staff there more intimately than I knew many of the attendings when I was an intern. The network also does a great job with translations. I don't know Portuguese, but I can interact in either English or Spanish because the system turns my words into language the Brazilians understand.

I know that this information technology underpinning my practice isn't something you think about. *Virtual reality* is not even in your vocabulary because the concept has become so common that it is transparent. Ironically, the term did not yet exist when I turned twenty-one, but it has come and gone in the nearly thirty years between our respective celebrations of this milestone birthday. "Old" folks like me are still awed by the evolution of telemedicine's ability to replicate virtually any clinical indicator and make it seem as real as something physically present—even though the patient may be elsewhere in time and/or space. I am equally impressed with how well we have learned to convey healing power over virtual networks. Early critics failed to see how well the art of medicine would adapt to the technology of telemedicine.

Just try to imagine the situation at the time of your birth when surgeons did not yet have the benefit of virtual construction from digitized diagnostic images. They could not practice the procedure to be performed on each patient before the actual operation. Surgeons back then might be compared to musicians who could not practice a piece until the public performance. In retrospect, how terrifying the medical world was when I entered it back in the late twentieth century!

Today, I can be sure that the surgeon who works on my patient has gotten all the practice she needs on the virtual case. My job is to be sure the surgical technician properly preps the patient in my office's telesurgical suite. The surgeon then performs the operation remotely, from his or her office or home, sending and receiving the data needed over the Universal Wide-Band ComNet. You may not believe this, but the surgeon and the patient always had to be in the same room at the same time back when you were born.

So, do you still want to be a doctor? If you are good enough, you may still want to consider becoming a professional cellist. A computer may produce the sound of your cello, but the computer will never capture the human feeling that you can give to Dvorak or Bach. Of course, neither is a computer capable of duplicating the feeling that can exist between doctor and patient when both are communicating on a human level.

One of my European colleagues on the Brazil project recently quoted a famous twentieth century Spanish endocrinologist and historian, Gregorio Marañón. "No hay enfermedades, sino enfermos." ("There are no such things as diseases, only sick people.") The project's computer can translate these words as well as I can, but it couldn't have written them—and it certainly cannot know what they really mean. I understand them. The difference between the computer and me comes back to what my father told me. The heart of the matter is the privilege of being let into your patients' lives so you can really help them.

I still love being a doctor, even though communications technology and computers have changed virtually every aspect of day-to-day practice since I started way back in the 1990s. Despite these changes, medicine has allowed me to make a living, to raise my kids in a small town, and to help a lot of people by practicing state-of-the-art medicine. Because of these changes, I am actively helping to eradicate an exotic disease in South America and giving my local patients direct access to the best diagnostic and therapeutic resources in the world, right in my office or in their homes.

I feel part of a world of healers. I think my patients do, too. We all have the continuous support, literally and virtually, of the whole world of medical knowledge. The telemedicine revolution that started to blossom around the time of your birth in 1999 has empowered healer and patient alike in surprising ways. Healthcare has never been the same since this revolution . . . and it has never been better.

I must quit now. I haven't used a keyboard for so long that my hands are starting to hurt. (There's one advantage to old technology. I'm sure I would say even more if I were dictating this to my computer as usual.) Best wishes on your twenty-first birthday. Rest assured that the future has more possibilities than you can possibly imagine. Being in the health professions is a great way to experience them.

Love from the digital dinosaur doctor,

3

CHAPTER

Of Images, Communications, and Technological Revolutions

Healthcare, attending to illness or injury and keeping people well, is a distinguishing characteristic of human beings. It crosses all cultures and times. Along with other fundamental human activities, medical science is one of the common denominators in our intellectual efforts to understand what happened and why. The evolution of many societies throughout archeological and recorded time is explained to some extent by their abilities to respond to a dangerous disease, a dysfunctional behavior, a tainted food supply, or a prevalent physical trauma.

Technology—often characterized as the realm of tools that translate scientific knowledge into useful activity—is another uniquely human endeavor. It also helps explain our past. Technology has rather regularly differentiated the victors from the vanquished and the haves from the have-nots. In healthcare, technology has been employed over time to generate the images that define illness or injury and guide healers in their interventions. Its evolution can be traced from prehistoric healing rituals depicted on cave walls with daubs of hand-ground pigment to today's computer-generated human genome maps projected from virtual space by an electron gun onto a phosphor-coated monitor screen.

Millions of images along the way, based on the latest technology of the day, record the history of medicine. These evolving images reflect the constant pursuit of new techniques to master the art and science of caring for our bodies and minds. However, the existence of images is not enough to explain changes in healthcare. Even a good image doesn't do much good if it exists in only one place. Expansion of a medical concept in space and time requires proliferation of the image.

Therefore, the communication of images and related explanatory information is another significant feature of the history of healthcare. (Indeed, more than a few medical discoveries and their related images have likely been lost over time simply because they were not communicated.) Knowing something about the possibilities for reproducing and distributing images greatly aids our understanding of the past and our insight into the future. By extension, the power of a potential change in healthcare is likely to be a direct function of the ease with which it can be communicated.

We have every reason to believe that the history of healthcare will continue to evolve with the production and communication of new images, just as it has in the past. However, a review of the history of healthcare shows that the changes are not always gradual. Every so often a new combination of technology and image is communicated so widely and so fast that it brings dramatic change. Telemedicine is poised to become one of those joint forces that revolutionizes healthcare. As a prelude to a practical and in-depth examination of the issues surrounding telemedicine, this chapter explains why telemedicine deserves to be taken seriously.

TELEMEDICINE IS . . . THE PERSONAL COMMUNICATIONS SYSTEM

Anyone who spends much time in a hospital has probably resented the incessant noise of the paging system (e.g., "Dr. Jones, please call extension 4177") or pondered the inefficiency of bedside buzzers that occasionally summon a nurse—and then come to the inevitable conclusion that there's got to be a better way to reach needed caregivers. How else could health professionals be contacted when they are out of hearing distance or away from the nurses' station?

Telemedicine provides an answer in the form of personal communications systems (PCS). Resulting from the convergence of wireless telephony and computer technologies, a PCS unit looks and works like a cellular telephone, but with added functions like pager and voice mail. Doctors and nurses can answer a call or page based on a specific cue (e.g., the unit shakes and rings if the message is urgent), or listen to voice mail when not otherwise occupied.

PCS frequently eliminates the need for face-to-face contact because so many problems can be quickly resolved over the telephone. The old way, buzzers and P.A.

COMMUNICATIONS

Telemedicine's vast potential is made possible by the unprecedented expansion in communications that has been a defining feature of the final years of the twentieth century. Never before has the world experienced such dramatic increases in the number of ways that information can be conveyed from one point to another, and telemedicine will undoubtedly take advantage of them all (albeit to varying degrees). Because reviews of specific communications technologies occur throughout this book, only a few comments are needed here to set the tone for subsequent discussion.

As recently as the early 1980s, almost all voice communications transpired over copper wires owned by the telephone monopoly (commonly referred to as Ma Bell) or radio waves. Both channels were heavily regulated by the Federal Communications Commission (FCC), state Public Utilities Commissions, or other government agencies. The telegram, a once popular alternative to telephone calls or letters, was used for little more than transferring money to distant relatives, sending brief greetings on special occasions, or tersely expressing opinions to members of Congress.[1] Printed communications were carried from sender to recipient almost entirely by U. S. Postal Service employees, bicycle couriers, or newspaper carriers. Television programming was basically run by three look-alike networks. This overall state of affairs in communications in the early 1980s had been relatively stable since the 1950s.

pages, wasted lots of time in comparison. PCS also allows caregivers to conduct verbal business while they are traveling between home, office, and hospital, and the communications can be easily encrypted to ensure confidentiality.

The revolution will be extended over the next few years when PCS and PDA (personal digital assistants, which are small computers like the Palm Pilot) become available in a single handheld unit—a great example of convergence. The Department of Defense has already deployed such integrated modules into daily healthcare operations with considerable success. Furthermore, military-funded research has produced several software packages to link PCS with laptop or desktop computers and networks.

Health professionals with PCS will have all needed information and contacts at their fingertips, literally, in the very near future. This technology will create unprecedented improvements in cost, quality, and access. It will also eliminate practitioners' well-worn excuse that they didn't get the message.

The number of changes occurring since the mid-1980s is truly re-markable in comparison. Cable television has grown from a few chan-nels of movies and sporting events to become the principal source of news and entertainment in the majority of American homes. Communications satellites now cover the globe at all hours from high, medium, and low orbits. Some of their signals are beamed to home satellite dishes—at first awkwardly large, now unobtrusively small—that have sprung up in backyards and on high-rise balconies all over the country. Fiberoptic cable has been strung from coast to coast and across borders. At the same time, the technology of wireless telephony has evolved so fast that some of the recently installed cable may never be used for its originally intended purpose.

Last, and definitely not least, the Internet and World Wide Web are changing just about everything—healthcare included—at warp speed. These telecomputing networks have given new meaning to the established concept of the Global Village, allowing multichannel com-munications in real-time all over the world and changing long-standing relationships in the process. Thomas L. Friedman, foreign af-fairs columnist for *The New York Times,* has aptly placed the Internet's impact in the broader context of recent world history:

> If all the threats and opportunities of the cold-war system grew out of "division," all the threats and opportunities of the globalization system grow out of "integra-tion." The symbol of the cold-war system was a wall, which divided everyone. The symbol of the globalization system is the World Wide Web, which unites everyone. In the cold war we reached for the hot line between the White House and the Kremlin—a symbol that we were all divided but at least someone, the two super-powers, were in charge. In the era of globalization we reach for the Internet—a symbol that we are all connected but nobody is in charge.[2]

Later in this book we will show how analogous changes will occur in healthcare because the impact of communications-based globaliza-tion extends far beyond geopolitics. The key point here is that new communications technologies are high on the list of forces changing well-established features of our old, familiar world. Satellites, wireless telephones, and computer networks are creating new possibilities for defining and delivering information-intensive services like healthcare. Thanks to the new tools of communications, telemedicine will move our industry, too, from "division" to "integration."

IMAGES

An image is not just a physical representation of visual material. Indeed, this book would be doing a disservice to the full potential of telemedicine if its scope were limited to the electronic transmission of visual images. An image is a representation, literally and figuratively. It is part physical—the arrangement of ink particles on paper, the silver grains on an X-ray film, the energized pixels on a video terminal—and part perceptual. The letters on this page, for example, are set within the broad context of contemporary English, our backgrounds and education, interest in the subject of this book, and a host of other factors that bring meaning to what we authors present to readers with our words. Everyone will read the same words, but each reader will construct a unique personal image of our intended message.

When books and photographs were being widely disseminated for the first time in the sixteenth and nineteenth centuries respectively, they irrevocably changed how the world was perceived. Painting has played a similar role in reflecting and shaping world views for an even longer time. Over the next few years, telemedicine will bring similarly deep alterations to the perceptual context of medicine itself. These changes affect how we think about—and, ultimately, how we actually do—healthcare.[3]

As mental pictures, images are laden with meaning that can go far beyond visual representation.[4] They may convey auditory, tactile, olfactory, gustatory, kinesthetic, or even emotional perceptions. Technology also enhances the power of images—as evidenced by the recent evolution of multimedia presentations. To update an old saying, if a picture is worth a thousand words, then a picture accompanied with hypertext links and a sound file (e.g., a good Web page) must be worth several thousand.

If anyone doubts the growing impact of images reinforced by other sensory inputs, simply remember the powerful impressions created by George Lucas' original "Star Wars" trilogy when the movies appeared in theaters in 1978, 1980, and 1983. Their ability to blur the distinction between real action and special effects was unprecedented. Next, consider how the originals pale in comparison with today's digitally remastered, enhanced-sound versions of the same films seen in a modern cineplex. Consider also the very different experiences of watching "Star Wars" on a VHS cassette in the late 1980s on a twenty-one inch stereo television set and watching it today from DVD on a thirty-five inch home entertainment center with five-channel Dolby surround sound. Yes, technology has changed the overall image, even though the picture has remained the same.[5]

Telemedicine will quickly bring comparable differences to the world of healthcare. As telemedicine advances, it will incorporate more of our senses and change our expectations—just as the new, multimedia technology of images has changed what we expect in entertainment. Because it is developing in the environment of so many new possibilities, telemedicine is much more than a new way to acquire, organize, transmit, and interpret the same old images of illness and injury. Telemedicine will give us new images in almost every aspect of healthcare, from underlying concepts of disease to organization of the delivery system.

LESSONS FROM THE INDUSTRIAL REVOLUTION

History has been shaped many times by technological revolutions. The development of metal tools, armaments and gunpowder, agricultural equipment, the printing press, and the steam engine all created relatively sudden and universal changes in the course of human affairs. The revolutions associated with these major developments have generally tended to occur several centuries apart, so relatively few generations actually know the transitional excitement of the revolutions themselves.

People living at the beginning of the twenty-first century will experience both the old and the new. We are the generation bridging the end of the Industrial Revolution and the beginning of the Information Revolution, and telemedicine is arriving on the scene at the time of a technological shift of seismic significance. A brief review of both revolutions is, therefore, needed to complete our description of the broad historical context against which telemedicine must be interpreted and understood.

The lessons to be learned are as much about new ways of organizing and perceiving as they are about the transformational tools

---

TELEMEDICINE IS . . . BABY PICTURES

A few years ago, a cartoon commentary on the incipient information revolution made the fax machine rounds. The drawing depicted a sign, festooned with balloons and ribbons, in front of a suburban home. The sign said, "It's a girl. Pictures available on our Website."

That cartoon turned out to be prophetic. With ever-wider access to the Internet and inexpensive digital cameras, more people are putting more personal things on Websites, including baby pictures. Now a health system—Scottsdale Healthcare in Shea and Osborn, Arizona—is posting pictures for the parents.

Since early 1998, the hospital has maintained an "on-line nursery" at its Website. After obtaining parents' permission, obstetrics nurses use a digital camera to snap

themselves. History shows time and again that new tools, after their introduction, become facilitators of the next shifts in perception and organization. The pace of this recursive process, one of change producing even more change, seems to accelerate with each succeeding revolution. Today's electronic tools are transforming lives much faster than a steam engine ever did. We can draw useful lessons from the previous revolutions, but we must not assume that they occur at the same rate. Indeed, speed is probably one of the defining differences between the Industrial and Information Revolutions. Information is faster.

Still, the Industrial Revolution marks the beginning of the modern age. It was not merely an economic revolution, initiating a new way of organizing production. It also marked the culmination of philosophical, religious, political, and social changes which had been brewing since the late Middle Ages. Democracy, free will, reason, and science gradually replaced church and king as the sources of knowledge and authority.

Within this new environment and with these new tools, an entrepreneurial middle class grew to develop the machines—first powered by water, then by coal and steam, and finally by electricity—that exponentially increased the output of material goods. The rest, as they say, is history, but a review of key events reveals an underlying social dynamism that will surely continue in the Information Revolution. In the next few pages we summarize the considerable extent to which a technology-based revolution can transform society.

Standardization, such as the interchangeable musket parts turned out at Eli Whitney's Connecticut factory beginning in 1798, laid the foundation for mass production. The technique was perfected with the moving assembly line, first used to manufacture the

pictures of newborns and any desired combinations of family members. Parents preview the photos and decide which ones they want to represent their recently-enlarged family to the electronic universe. The selected images, a short message from the parents, baby weight, length, hair and eye color, and delivering physician's name are all posted on the site. For security purposes, only first names are used.

Friends and relatives who have access to the Internet can check out the new kids and their families from anywhere in the world. The files are left on-line as long as the hospital's server disk space allows. Along with their baby, parents may take home a floppy disk with all the picture files.

Needless to say, the site is full of images of the cutest babies in the world. Just ask their parents. You can visit the on-line nursery at www.shc.org.

PIONEERS IN TELEMEDICINE: ACE ALLEN, M.D.

The clicking sound of his computer keyboard was heard frequently during the course of our telephone interview with Ace Allen, M.D. He was looking things up as questions arose during our conversation and sending us E-mails about resources he thought could be useful in writing this book. But he never seemed distracted. Ace used the information that he made appear on his monitor to add depth to our dialogue. Technophilia—dating back to his first computer, an Apple II he purchased in 1980—is his means, and communication is the end.

Communication is the common thread in all of Ace Allen's interests, including medicine. He spent the first seven years of his medical career as an oncologist, a subspecialty noted for the intensity of feelings that are aroused when patients and families face cancer. The one thing he truly misses since he gave up practice in 1995 is the "I-Thou nature of patient care."

Cancer prevention and early intervention were the passions of Dr. Allen's oncology career. Telemedicine turned out to be a logical way to marry his need to communicate with his interest in bringing services to cancer patients earlier in the course of the disease.

One of his duties as an assistant professor of medicine at the University of Kansas, located in Kansas City, was to staff outreach oncology clinics in Hays, Kansas, over 250 miles to the west. Several times in the winter of 1991-1992, "big Midwest weather" made travel impossible, forcing cancellation of the clinic. Dr. Robert Cox, a Hays pediatrician (see profile on page 64 and 65), had an established interactive video link to the university that they had been using to deliver pediatric subspecialty clinics. Instead of canceling his clinics, Dr. Allen employed the system to bring high-powered oncology consultation to thirty patients on the distant storm-bound prairie.

Dr. Allen surveyed the patients and physicians who had participated in these clinics and found high levels of satisfaction among them. "That's when I decided telemedicine was what I wanted to do." His resumé shows a sharp discontinuity. Before 1992 Dr. Allen published articles on chemotherapy, smoking cessation, and reports of unusual cancer cases. Afterward, the published articles are on telemedicine.

In 1993, Ace received a Career Development Award from the Department of Prevention and Control of the National Cancer Institute.

One of the goals of the grant was to improve patient access to high-quality services. Evaluation data subsequently showed that, over the project's five years, telemedicine had shortened the time to diagnosis and treatment in cancer patients over a wide swath of rural Kansas by providing access to better, more consistent care.

Dr. Allen has been working since 1995 on applying telemedicine to home care which, he says, "is the most natural area for cost/benefit besides prison care." He helped develop a program in Lawrence, Kansas that provides a video connection between clients and providers via the local cable television system. Based on his data, Ace estimates that half of the 1.5 million daily home care visits made in the United States could be accomplished by telemedicine, at a cost of $15–20 per visit, versus $95 for an in-person contact. In 1999, a two-way video connection over telephone lines can be installed in a home for $500.

Here's a perfectly feasible use of telemedicine that could save billions of dollars. Yet it hasn't taken off. The reason, says Dr. Allen, is the current unhappy state of the politics and economics of federally funded home healthcare.

Politics, organization, and human factors—not technology—are the usual reasons for failure of telemedicine systems. Critical factors for success include how needs are identified, who is brought into the planning process, and where the financial incentives are placed. Many telemedicine programs have been underutilized because they were designed from the top down to chase federal dollars, rather than to meet a real need. Dr. Allen observes, "There is a predictable inverse relationship between federal funding and clinical use of a system."

Ace distills what he has learned about the adoption of electronic technology in medicine to two principles: "If it doesn't make the practitioner's life easier it won't be adopted, no matter what it does" and "Any change in the technical environment of medicine will necessitate an equal or greater change in the operational environment." In other words, change is hard, which is why he predicts gradual adoption of telemedicine rather than revolutionary restructuring. He holds his forecasts to a minimum. "I keep a crystal ball in my office to remind us that you can drop it at any time."

Currently, Ace's main job is as editor of *Telemedicine Today,* one of the foremost publications in the field. He continues researching, writing, consulting, and speaking. Communication is still his thing. Technology extends his reach and power.

Model-T automobile in 1914. With that product, Henry Ford realized his dream of creating "a car for the great multitude," which, he said, could be purchased in any color, as long as it was black. By the early 1920s, harnessing the power of mass production at such facilities as the 80,000 worker River Rouge plant, Ford was able to produce 60 percent of the automobiles marketed in the United States while paying its workers an unprecedented $5 per day.

The industrial enterprise was organized to produce and market larger and larger quantities of goods. Corporations grew nationally and internationally to exploit economies of scale. By the first two decades of the twentieth century, corporate giants such as Standard Oil, Carnegie Steel, Union Pacific Railroad, Ford, and Sears-Roebuck, had staked out enormous territories in the economic landscape. Their models of mass production and mass marketing had become the dominant paradigm for doing business in America and Europe.

Management science and communications technologies were spawned to serve the needs of companies that were growing in size and spreading throughout the world. This time period also saw the rise of universal public education because industrialization required hosts of managers, scientists, engineers, accountants, and other knowledge workers to make the enterprise run.

The Industrial Revolution created rising economic expectations. Average workers aspired to own their own homes and to purchase a host of consumer goods. Economic downturns and wars periodically slowed—but could not reverse—the overall trend toward economic prosperity. The consumption society continued to grow. Magazines were published and distributed nationally. Sears Roebuck did coast-to-coast business via its local stores and its famous catalog.

TELEMEDICINE IS . . . COMPREHENSIVE DENTAL CARE

Teledentistry might seem a bit implausible. After all, how could we possibly get a filling or a cleaning without sitting in the dentist's chair? Telemedicine's contributions to dentistry will come in other ways for the foreseeable future, but they will greatly improve the efficiency and effectiveness of our dental care.

One significant gain is the general or family dentist's ability to get a specialist's opinion without sending the patient to the specialist. Without telemedicine, patients and their records are commonly sent to dental specialists (e.g., periodontists, orthodontists) for a consultative visit—with all the attendant hassles of making the extra appointment and taking time off from work. The specialist then examines the patient and sends a treatment recommendation back to the

Still, the mass market could not be fully exploited until new technology harnessed mass communications. Radio, and later television, could reach millions simultaneously with the same message. With mass media, pitches for products could be brought into virtually every living room in America. The location of those living rooms changed, too. Fewer farmers were needed to produce food and fibers, and more workers were needed in factories. Industrialization created urbanization.

Industrialization also changed healthcare. Since medicine largely reflects the society it serves, American medicine became technology-oriented, urban-focused, centralized, hierarchical, and bureaucratic. The industry quickly learned how to meet consumers' insatiable demands fueled by the rapid rise of health insurance in the two decades following World War II. It also succeeded in keeping people alive longer.

Not only did medicine's curative powers grow tremendously from the beginning to the end of the Industrial Revolution, but healthcare grew from insignificance to become one of the largest sectors in the American economy. This growth has been accompanied in recent decades by considerable anxiety about the costs of care and has raised profound issues about the allocation of medical resources. The ensuing economic, political, and social questions are not the subject of this book, but telemedicine will change the answers in the twenty-first century. The subject of this book is how telemedicine will offer many new possibilities for improving efficiency, effectiveness, equity, quality, access, and cost.

As noted previously in this chapter, much of human history is explained in the context of revolutionary technological changes, and the rate of recursive change seems to be accelerating. Therefore, we should not be surprised that urbanization, workplace hierarchy, economies of

---

referring dentist. With telemedicine, the referring dentist can instead send high-resolution intraoral pictures, X rays, and other dental records. The patient is spared the inconvenience of the extra trip to the specialist's office, and possibly the expense of the consultation.

The quality of overall patient care will also be enhanced by telemedicine as dentists begin using the new technologies to confer with other practitioners. In particular, dentists and physicians can establish electronic links that will allow both to deliver more comprehensive care. A dentist could get a physician to review intraoral pictures of a lesion that might be a sign of serious systemic disease, and a physician could get a dentist to review digitized pictures and other records to help diagnose a patient's facial swelling or head and neck pain. Indeed, inter-professional contacts may be a great growth area for telemedicine.

scale, mass marketing, and other features of the Industrial Revolution are already giving way to a rural renaissance, collaborative work arrangements, artisanal products, individualized media, and a new consumerism. As it has over the past two hundred years, healthcare is changing in parallel to society's changes. Mediated by telemedicine, the coming changes will be extraordinary.

THE PROMISE OF THE INFORMATION REVOLUTION

Historians disagree about the beginning of the Industrial Revolution. Some say it began with the exploitation of steam power by the Newcomen siphon engine in 1712; others date it from Watt's invention of the steam condenser engine in 1763. Identifying the arrival of the Information Revolution is a bit easier.

The first electronic digital computer, named ENIAC (an acronym for Electronic Numerical Integrator and Computer), began its work in 1943 at the University of Pennsylvania by computing artillery shell trajectories for the U.S. Army. The computing machine weighed thirty tons and filled a two-story, thirty foot by fifty foot room with 18,000 vacuum tubes and countless resistors, capacitors, and wires. ENIAC consumed so much electricity that the lights of Philadelphia reportedly dimmed when it was first switched on. It cost nearly a half million dollars to build. Even though it had less processing power than a handheld calculator available today for less than $20, it was a computer—the first general purpose electronic digital computing device ever.

This big clunker did not initially inspire contemporaries to wax poetic about the coming Information Revolution. Thomas J. Watson, Sr., President of IBM, is reputed to have said in 1949 that the world would someday need about a dozen such computers. But thanks to subsequent development of the transistor and integrated circuits printed on little wafers of silicon, computers have become faster, smaller, cheaper, and more reliable. The pronouncement of Moore's Law in 1965 formally recognized the fact that a revolution was occurring in our ability to process information.

Gordon Moore, then chairman of Intel (still the world's largest manufacturer of computer chips), observed that the amount of random access memory available per square inch on a single silicon chip was doubling about every eighteen months. Random access memory (called RAM) is effectively the horsepower of computing. It is one of the key factors that defines the power and performance capabilities of a system. Increasing density of RAM chips has generally been accompanied by manufacturing efficiencies, consistently allowing prices to fall while performance rises. Nothing else in the history of human technology has come vaguely close to matching this rate of improvement in performance.

Rapid progress in computing power was initially evident in the growth of large mainframe computers. Almost all major businesses, including hospitals and health insurance companies, had installed mainframes by the end of the 1970s. However, the principal product of mainframes was printouts—endless reams of paper that did little more than compile existing information from numerous sources into one paper document. Such automation was impressive at the time, but it wasn't enough to revolutionize a business or industry.

Really meaningful changes began to occur when the computer moved from mainframes the size of upright freezers (usually stored in controlled-access, air-conditioned rooms) to small "desktop" computers in the early 1980s. When networks began to link desktop units to other computers, the flow of information in an enterprise could become nearly frictionless. One of the simplest examples of the power of networking is the cash register that reads bar codes. While human checkers collect money for goods purchased, the network ties together the company's computers (some disguised as cash registers) and keeps track of inventory, sends up-to-the-minute information on store performance to the desktop computers of local and regional managers, and orders replacement stock.

Networked information processing can provide widespread access to virtually any information needed to write a contract, service a customer, expedite a shipment, run a company, or care for a patient. Information-empowered employees distribute the administrative burden and flatten the hierarchy. But what does this mean to customers (still widely known as patients in the health industry)?

Employees empowered by computer networks can serve customers more nimbly. The company is no longer so dependent on centralized oversight to keep things coordinated. A relatively independent staff can work with customers to meet their needs and simultaneously keep the enterprise informed of all relevant activity. Information-savvy service businesses in the 1990s have streamlined functions such as airline booking and insurance claims processing by giving their customer service representatives, via a computer, all the information they need to handle the whole transaction. The next step, already well under way in many businesses, is giving the customer direct access to the computer. (As will be shown in subsequent chapters, this step hints of several ways that telemedicine will free traditional medical care of the constraints of space and time.)

Networked computers are facilitating work reengineering, too. In hospitals, for example, job classifications are converging as clerks and clinical people work together on the ward to care for patients without having to turn to the business office, respiratory care service, or patient transportation department. Their computers allow them to register the patient, order and document treatments, and coordinate X-ray studies from the nurses' station or even the bedside. Less time is spent shuffling papers, making phone calls, and transporting patients.

Because fewer people need to interact with each patient and those who do are occupied by less red tape, frontline workers actually have enhanced opportunity to be at the bedside with patients, getting to know them and their problems and needs. Patient focus ("customer focus" in the business world) is facilitated. Any business using these techniques has the makings of excellence, in the best Tom Peters[6] sense of the word.

The Information Revolution has affected manufacturing as much as it has changed service businesses. Modern ideas of quality control, developed by Deming and Juran in the mid-twentieth century, are based on using information to control industrial processes. Adopted by the Japanese after World War II, these techniques account in large measure for the success of the modern Japanese economy.

TELEMEDICINE IS . . . A RURAL COMMUNITY HEALTH INFORMATION NETWORK

The conventional image of telemedicine is interactive video linking a rural patient and doctor with medical specialists at an urban health center. Franklin Memorial Hospital in Farmington, Maine, was one of the country's first small hospitals to install a video link back in the 1970s in partnership with local physicians, but it has recently developed much richer applications of telemedicine.

Concerned about the future of rural hospitals, residents of west central Maine held a series of well-attended health summits beginning in 1994 to define a viable vision for local healthcare. Citizens from many different backgrounds (e.g., education, banking, manufacturing) joined healthcare leaders in identifying the area's unmet health needs and exploring how new technologies could help solve problems. The result was the creation of a new parent organization, Franklin Community Health Network, and the creation of new affiliates for primary care, mental health, and community education and outreach.

The Network established an on-line presence (http://www.fchn.org) in 1997. Local citizens can visit this rapidly growing, well-maintained Website to access hundreds of resources on topics like aging, mental health, wellness, nutrition, and smoking cessation. They can check the credentials and hospital privileges of local

The core concept in contemporary quality control is that information about a process must be fed back and applied continuously to improve that process. On the production line, it replaces the concepts of Taylorism,[7] the turn-of-the century mass production ideal of a worker who is as machine-like as possible. In the information age, all movements do not need to be scripted and controlled by an efficiency expert. Production workers become more than a set of hands. They are crucial links in the process, constantly assessing how things are going, making adjustments, informing others, suggesting changes in the process, and sometimes even stopping the whole production line when things have gone too far awry. Such thinking could not have occurred during the Industrial Revolution.

In the last decade, healthcare institutions have begun implementing information-based concepts of quality control. For example, studies have targeted hospital length-of-stay of pneumonia patients, readmission rates of heart failure patients, blood sugar levels of diabetics, or patients' satisfaction with the food service. The outcome data are continuously fed back into the information system, using standard quality improvement tools, to make the process better. Accurate and timely information is obviously crucial to the success of these projects. An electronic network can greatly facilitate collecting, processing, and distributing that information.

doctors, explore payment options and programs for patients who cannot afford to pay, or identify a support group. Residents of outlying communities can determine the next time the mobile health unit will be in their "neck of the woods" (a phrase with literal meaning in western Maine).

The Website also supports recruiting for the system by posting current job openings and information about the region. Local practitioners can benefit by accessing a special site (http://www.fchn.org/dochome.htm) that connects them with national data banks of medical information. The Network is currently bringing all physicians in the service area on-line (providing equipment if needed), so every practitioner in the area will soon have access to the most up-to-date technical information.

A wallet-size plastic Health Card encoded with personal health information has been given to almost all 40,000 residents of the Network's service area. This smart card is the foundation for a database that will be used in many ways to track and improve health in the community. Ultimately, network technologies will link databases, technical resources, consumer health information, provider guidelines, and electronic medical records. Although the original interactive video link is seldom used these days, the citizens of west central Maine are well on their way to establishing the new, expanded benchmark for rural telemedicine.

The industrial age's assembly line—useful when the objective was to produce huge quantities of invariant products—is being superseded in the information age by integrated, interacting, flexible teams that work together to produce smaller lots of customized goods and solve problems along the way. Thanks to the Information Revolution, manufacturing is becoming smaller scale, more flexible, and customized. The success of this new model is largely due to networked computers, with their ability to connect everybody, from customer to shop worker. This higher level of interpersonal connection is having a huge effect on healthcare, one of our economy's most individualized businesses. Communications technology increasingly allows healthcare providers and practitioners to serve individual patients locally with customized, state-of-the-art healthcare products in a larger, geographically diverse healthcare system.

How businesses communicate with customers has also changed as a result of the Information Revolution. To understand the extent and nature of these changes, think about the mail you have received over the past week. How many different catalogs did you get? How many fund-raising letters came your way? How many magazines sent you subscription solicitations? Most of the mailings were probably relevant to you and your tastes in some way because mail is often targeted directly by marketers who use computers to "mine" massive databases of information about regions, census tracts, and individual customers. They can learn much about you by examining your past spending patterns, for example, and then target you for specialty magazines filled with advertising aimed at people like you.

Even on television, with the abundance of offerings available via cable system or satellite dish, you typically sample a unique personal mix of programming with the help of a remote control. You wind up seeing programs that the TV industry is trying to match with people like you. So many choices are available because producers and executives have enough information to isolate an increasing number of smaller-but-profitable markets, based on all our differences. Compare this evolving state of affairs with American traditions like the annual Sears catalog that used to be a fixture in virtually every American household[8] or the three television networks that ruled the airways for so long.

"One size fits all" doesn't work any more. The mature processes of the Industrial Revolution—mass production, mass media, mass marketing, and mass society—are all in decline as a result of the Information Revolution. Can the traditional ways of "mass medicine" be far behind? The good news is that the Information Revolution provides tools for creating different-but-desirable alternatives in virtually every realm of our personal and professional lives, including healthcare.

Internet-based "push" technologies, individually tailored to bring just the right information to each customer, and "pull" technologies, allowing consumers to find the information that they want when they want it, are growing at a phenomenal rate in all fields. Specialized software packages, known as intelligent agents, that are user-programmed to search a network automatically and bring back information or complete transactions have already made their debut.

Just as the Industrial Revolution greatly diminished the role of heavy human labor by harnessing the power of machines to do the same work, the Information Revolution is using computer power to accomplish more and more tasks that had previously been done with paper and pencil. In today's economy, human workers will be increasingly valued for their abilities to understand and use information, to create new things, and interact empathetically with other people. These are the job skills that will be valued even more in the future, especially in healthcare. The patient-practitioner relationship and the healing that flows from it will not soon be usurped by machines.

Not only are manufacturing, design, marketing, and service functions devolving to smaller and different work groups. Thanks to the Information Revolution, these work groups are dispersing, too. Since organizations require less face-to-face and face-to-paper interaction, electronic communications—in the form of telephone, fax, E-mail, interactive conferencing, and a host of other technologies examined later in this book—can serve as the link that keeps people in the mainstream in both their work and personal lives. Healthcare institutions are becoming virtual organizations defined by common interests and tied together by electronic communications; they will not be defined by people working together in the same building at the same time.

More people are working at home, and they are making their homes in different places. The suburbanization that began in the 1950s as the result of mass-produced autos, freeways, and tract homes has given way to a renaissance of rural areas and center-cities as people learn that they can do their information-based work from anywhere. Thanks to the Information Revolution, the rural population is growing at a pace not seen since the closing of the frontier in the early 1900s. The forgotten downtown areas of many major cities, no longer subservient to declines in manufacturing, are also rebounding. Today, communities that were facing serious shortages of health professionals only ten years ago find themselves in a much better position to attract doctors and other practitioners.

PIONEERS IN TELEMEDICINE: MICHAEL CAPUTO

Michael Caputo went to college to be a photographer or filmmaker, majoring in photographic arts and sciences at the Rochester Institute of Technology. The first year of classes was heavy on the sciences, especially imaging technology. "I fell in love with the technology," he says, in a way which explains much of his success in telemedicine. He understands and loves the technology of imaging.

During college in the mid-1980s, Mike was invited to work at NASA as a summer student. He was assigned to the Medical Sciences Division, where he was given the task of devising a way to acquire digital video images directly through a light microscope. Previously, images were photographed on slide film that had to be developed and digitized before being analyzed or transmitted. This was a cumbersome and time-consuming process, especially for use in outer space where everything is measured in terms of time and payload.

The project was supposed to take all summer. His technological expertise enabled Caputo to cobble together lenses and video equipment that solved the problem in about a week. He was hired by a NASA contractor as soon as he graduated.

The next undertaking took several years. It involved video retinal imaging—a considerably more complex problem, principally because of limitation in the brightness of the light that can be shined into a living eye and because of the operator's need to look through the instrument while capturing images. Since 1992 the resulting system has been on eleven space shuttle missions, capturing 3-D images that reveal details such as retinal blood vessel caliber and optic nerve head elevation. Caputo not only designed the system, but he also trained the crews in using it and had a hand in analyzing the data.

The job in Houston lasted seven years, during which time Mike was involved in dozens of telemedicine and medical imaging projects. Meanwhile, he earned a master's degree in physiological optics from the University of Houston.

Inevitably, the military recognized the utility of some of Mike's inventions in locales less exotic than outer space. One collaborative project sponsored by the Department of Defense, for example, captured retinal images of thirty-six patients in Denver and transmitted them via NASA satellite to specialists in Houston. The project found 96 percent agreement between diagnoses made by remote ophthalmologists and those made by doctors who had examined the patients in person. What's more, the operators in Denver were non-ophthalmologists (including Caputo himself). The examiner in Houston directed the distant operator via audio link. With the favorable results of this project and other demonstrations of the validity of data collected remotely, the momentum for telemedicine built rapidly.

Though Caputo's career in Houston was going extremely well, when C. Everett Koop offered him a job in Hanover, New Hampshire, he couldn't turn it down. Caputo, born and raised in New Hampshire, was anxious to move closer to home. Dr. Koop hired him in 1994 to manage a new project, the Northern New England Health Informatics Initiative. Caputo's mission was to serve as an expert in implementing telemedicine projects in Maine, New Hampshire, and Vermont. With counsel from his Harvard MBA brother, Michael fulfilled his agreement with the Koop Institute by founding Medical Dynamics, a company that contracted with the Institute to provide expertise in everything from technology selection to operator training.

Currently, Caputo is Director of Telemedicine Operations at Fletcher Allen Hospital of the University of Vermont in Burlington. Eighteen sites are now operational—offering grand rounds, classes for health students, and active clinical consultation (especially in dermatology and surgery). An ongoing fee-for-service consultation link has been established with Argentina and explored with Vietnam.

His department has ambitious plans. The Healthcare Center has promised to invest $30 million in information technology, which will put a networked computer on the desktop of most physicians in Vermont.

Caputo feels that reimbursement for telemedicine services and licensing issues are the biggest obstacles to further development. The crucial technical concern is to apply the appropriate level of technology to solve each problem, which is what Caputo considers to be his greatest strength. Telemedicine must respond to established work patterns efficiently and cheaply. Transmission and reception should occur right from the exam room or home where the patient is—not from down the hall, and certainly not from across the street.

Michael Caputo does still own a camera and occasionally finds time to use it artistically. But most of his creative energy has remained focused on the technological side. "I have fun doing what I do. And there is a deep sense of satisfaction every time I see a telemedicine consult that actually helps a patient."

Just as the Industrial Revolution generated significant social and cultural changes, the Information Revolution is bringing changes that extend far beyond the usual confines of technology. The same computers that have reorganized our workplace and marketplace have nurtured the development of exciting new world views, including chaos theory and the cybernetics of self-organizing systems. Our leisure environments are being changed as much as our work sites. Art museums, concert halls, movie theaters, and amusement arcades are filled with images that are created and processed digitally. New methods for accessing incredible quantities of information have even created an eclectic post-modern aesthetic, including music that is constructed from samples of other works and hypertext-based literature that allows readers to create their own unique paths through a story.

Concepts of education and literacy are shifting, too. While some critics worry about how little children read, we nevertheless turn to our kids when we need help with our Internet connection. Our whole world is changing—not just the world, but the images we use to represent and understand it, and not just the images, but ourselves. Nothing will be the same as it was, especially healthcare. Telemedicine is a part of something big. It is the vehicle through which the Information Revolution will transform medicine.

NOTES

1. Perhaps symbolically, the death knell for telegraphy was sounded in 1998 when the use of Morse code was officially ended by the International Telecommunications Union. This event reminds us of ongoing technological progress because the telegraph was the major communications breakthrough of the nineteenth century. For a concise and interesting review of the history of the development of telegraphy and its inventors, see Tom Standage's *The Victorian Internet* (New York: Walker and Company, 1998).

2. Thomas L. Friedman. "A Manifesto for the Fast World," *The New York Times Magazine* (March 28, 1999) 42 (adapted from his book, *The Lexus and the Olive Tree: Understanding Globalization,* (New York: Farrar, Strauss & Giroux, 1999).

3. Marshall McLuhan is the commentator who has contributed most to raising our culture's consciousness of the interaction between communication medium and perception. His books, especially *The Medium is the Message* [McLuhan M, Q Fiore, and J Ayd. New York, Bantam, 1967] have had a huge influence on modern (some would say post-modern) thought.

4. Recognizing that not all our readers want or need an in-depth analysis of the fascinating history and meaning of images, we present just enough discussion here to establish the long-term importance of images in the specific context of telemedicine. Extensive and thought-provoking inquiries into the transformational power of images in a wide variety of areas can be found in Paul Levinson's *The Soft Edge: A Natural History and Future of the Information Revolution* (London and New York: Routledge, 1997) and Mitchell Stephens' *The Rise of the Image, The Fall of the Word* (New York: Oxford University Press, 1998).

5. According to Orville Schell's review of "The Phantom Menace," the mind-boggling advance in multisensory images apparently continues with the fourth "Star Wars" installment that appeared at about the time this chapter was being written. "As the viewer is veritably engulfed by spaceships streaking across the galaxy and strange new characters, the THX sound system makes the very darkness vibrate." (*The New York Times,* March 21, 1999, AR 29)

6. See Peters T and RH Waterman, *In Search of Excellence: Lessons from America's Best-Run Businesses* (New York: Harper and Row, 1982), and many subsequent writings by Tom Peters on the theme of excellence in business.

7. Taylorism gets its name from Frederick W. Taylor. His pioneering studies of workers at a steel mill analyzed how the most efficient workers did their jobs then applied that knowledge to job organization and training. Publication of his seminal work, *Principles of Scientific Management,* in 1910 was the beginning of the science of efficiency, based on a hierarchical model which sought the greatest efficiency by empowering managers to treat workers as cogs in a machine.

8. Even the venerable Sears catalog has split into a number of smaller publications targeted to specific audiences to sell baby clothes, sporting goods, furniture, or tools, for example.

4
CHAPTER

Medical Revolutions:
The First Six

---

rev•o•lu•tion

n: alteration or change in some matter or respect: as: a sudden, radical, or complete change <a ~ in thought; a basic reorientation and reorganization <a ~ in
technology>; *also:* the interval of time during which such a movement occurs

Webster's Third New International Dictionary[1]

Outsiders (and even some insiders) who are unfamiliar with the history of healthcare in the United States are surprised to learn that the
underlying fundamentals of medicine have changed rather often.
Contrary to the popular image of an innately human enterprise built
on an enduring foundation of scientific truth, the reality is that healthcare has been reoriented and reorganized many times because key
variables were suddenly, radically, or completely altered. According to
the dictionary definition just given, then, medicine is not immune to
revolutions. It is as susceptible to major change as any other enterprise mentioned in the previous chapter.

The changes that merit classification as revolutions can occur in
one or more areas. For example, a scientific discovery can completely
redefine the organizing concepts of health and disease. A shift in the
country's political or economic circumstances might disenfranchise a
large group of patients and bring others into the system. The methods
and locations of healthcare can be transformed within a matter of

months by a technological development. And educational reforms or shifts in market power can cause the qualifications for professional practice to be redefined.

Before identifying previous revolutions in the modern era of American medicine and exploring their implications for the future of healthcare in general and telemedicine in particular, a few words need to be said about a relevant concept from the history of science. Americans have become rather familiar with the concept of paradigm shift, and it is relevant here.

The General Concept of Paradigm Shifts

Though subject to occasional charges of superficiality and overuse, the concept of paradigm shift can, when carefully applied, shed useful light on our belief that the intersection of telecomputing technology and medical information is true revolution, one as important as any that has happened in the brief history of modern health care.[2] The idea was originally proposed in the late 1940s by Thomas S. Kuhn in the first draft of what was to become his masterwork as a science historian, *The Structure of Scientific Revolutions*.[3]

Kuhn's career focused on understanding the discontinuities in scientific thought that are generally referred to as revolutions, including such well-known examples as the transition from geocentric to heliocentric organization of the solar system, from classical to quantum description of atomic structure, from static to evolutionary biology of species, and from Newtonian to relativistic cosmology. Each shift represented a new way of conceptualizing and understanding an important aspect of the world—figuratively, a new world view.

Science generally tends to move forward in a gradual fashion, with information added bit by bit to the reigning theory by scientists who have all been trained in the same schools and studied the same textbooks. As they continue to construct their model, they occasionally encounter anomalous observations, little bits of data that are not easily explained by the conventional wisdom. The model of reality is adjusted and patched, the world view modified incrementally.

Occasionally and unpredictably (except in retrospect), along comes a new model—one which provides a compellingly different explanation for the data that were previously dismissed or clumsily incorporated into the old system. This new view of reality so challenges the assumptions of the prevailing model that it must be called revolutionary. It brings with it a whole new way of thinking and often causes the leading proponents of the established order to launch a protective counter-offensive. Eventually, the new paradigm becomes institutionalized in schools and textbooks, and the cycle continues.[4] Preservation of the cumulative pile of old viewpoints is relegated to historians.

Even the concept of paradigm shifts is subject to challenge. One of the most widely respected physicists of the twentieth century, Freeman J. Dyson, has not only argued that modern interpretations of Kuhn's work are wrong, but also that Kuhn himself renounced the prevailing view of Kuhnian thinking shortly before his death in 1996.[5] Dyson argues instead that new technologies and tools, not new ideas and paradigms, explain scientific progress.[6]

Since we believe that new technologies and new ideas are working synergistically to revolutionize medicine and healthcare, we are not bothered by the ultimate outcome of this debate. Indeed, the dictionary definition at the beginning of this chapter includes both thought and technology within the scope of revolution. Kuhn and Dyson can both be right. (If you are confused, you get the point. Today's world *is* confusing.)

Paradigm Shifts in Modern Medicine and Healthcare

We admit at the outset that several dimensions of our seven-revolution model of medical paradigm shifts are arbitrary.

- We could have started at an earlier point in time if we had wanted to extend our scope beyond the modern era of medicine.
- We could have started at a later point in time by choosing an alternate definition of the modern era.
- We could have elevated some significant events, such as the rapid growth of health insurance in the two decades following World War II, to revolutionary status.
- We could have combined a few of our designated revolutions, such as the scientific development of a disease model and Flexner-era educational reform.

However, for a variety of reasons, we did not. We considered alternate designations that would have lengthened the list and others that would have made it shorter. (The average number of designations came out to around seven, any way we made the cut.) In the final analysis, we make no apologies for our final list of revolutions because this book is about the future of medicine, not its past.[7] Anyone who wants to quibble about our selection of specific paradigm shifts may have a good historical point, but they would be missing our future-focused points that some changes are bigger than others and that the new development we are considering—telemedicine—ranks with the biggest of them from the past.[8] According to the dictionary definition, it qualifies as a revolution on both counts, thought and technology. Telemedicine is not only the application of a new technology, but also the basis of a new way of thinking about the problems and prospects of human health.

REVOLUTION #1: ANESTHESIA

The development of anesthesia during the 1840s was hardly the first major change in the history of human healthcare, but it is often identified as the advance that launched the modern era of medical practice. Indeed, prior to the discovery of ether anesthesia in 1846, surgery in the United States had a decidedly negative image. Medical care and its practitioners were anything but respected or respectable:

> At the time, the public, understandably, held the medical profession in low esteem. Treatments were often unpleasant and their outcomes doubtfully effective.[9]

Early nineteenth century doctors were making considerable progress in their knowledge of anatomy and their ability to remove or repair dysfunctional human tissues, but the public's willingness to submit to their surgical interventions was dramatically diminished by fear of pain. The common phrase, "bite the bullet," is a literal reminder of the pre-anesthesia days when patients had to be forcibly engaged in

---

TELEMEDICINE IS . . . THE ELECTRONIC CURBSIDE CONSULT

When you interview physicians about where they get medical information, they will tell you they read reputable journals and look things up in books. When you actually follow them around, you find that they get much of their day-to-day help in making patient care decisions by "curbside consult," the term used for informal consultation with colleagues. Asking the right question of the right person is usually the best way to get the help a doctor needs to manage a patient problem. Any competent practicing physician will have cultivated a network of experts who can be consulted with the ease of a phone call.

Because of the specificity of the information elicited, phone consultation is a relatively efficient way to gather information. That is, it would be efficient if it weren't for telephone tag, a frustrating and time-wasting game that seems to have been made even worse by the pervasiveness of answering machines and voice mail.

Now, thanks to a service developed by George Bergus, M.D., Associate Professor of Family Medicine at the University of Iowa Hospitals and Clinics, some family doctors throughout that state play a lot less phone tag by taking advantage of E-mail consultation. The store-and-forward nature of that medium—allowing messages to be sent, picked up, and answered at any time—means no more waiting on hold, navigating voice mail mazes, or exchanging messages that boil down to "you're it."

other activity to distract them from the pain inflicted by surgery. As further evidence of the fear of premodern medicine, we have many old Western movies that depict a bunch of cowboys restraining a struggling patient (generally after priming him with whiskey) while the frontier doctor removes a bullet and closes the wound.

The discovery of ether as a potentially safe remedy to the pain problem did not immediately improve the image of medicine. Much experimentation and many years of practice by nurses, physicians, and dentists were ultimately needed to master the safe administration of ether and the other early anesthetic agents. Nevertheless, health professionals were able to begin reorienting their public image and changing their practices when they learned how to control pain. This is much more than a minor adjustment in the course of healthcare; it is the revolution that provided the foundation of respectability on which healthcare has grown ever since.

REVOLUTION #2: SCIENTIFIC DISEASE MODEL AND PUBLIC HEALTH

Anesthesia established the foundation for public trust in healthcare by overcoming one of its most unpleasant aspects, pain, but it did not solve the equally vexing problem of doubtful effectiveness. In other

Family doctors at University of Iowa-affiliated clinics were the initial beneficiaries of the E-mail Consult Service (ECS), which allows them to send queries to twenty-nine subspecialists at the University and receive a response within a day. The ECS has recently been extended to graduates of the residency who have remained in Iowa, and to physicians at eight family practice residency programs throughout the state.

To maintain confidentiality, patient-identifying data are left off all queries, and messages are encrypted before being transmitted. Most questions are answered within twelve hours, 98 percent of them by E-mail. The system archives all queries and responses and makes them available to all system users. Family doctors have found this database of questions asked by their peers to be a rich information resource in itself. The accumulated data might also be used for research into the consultation patterns of family doctors, as well as to plan continuing medical education.

The family physicians who use ECS are unanimous in their love for it. Eighty percent of the consultants admit that they like it, too, finding that the E-mail is easy to integrate into their daily routine. None feel they have lost patients by participating, and several consultants believe that ECS has led to increased referrals. Above all, nobody misses telephone tag.

PIONEERS IN TELEMEDICINE: ROBERT COX, M.D.

"I'm an introvert except when it comes to telemedicine. It's my 'hot button,'" says Dr. Robert Cox, M.D. He has no doubt that his work in telemedicine will have a far greater positive impact on health, especially of rural people, than anything he could do seeing one patient at a time.

Dr. Cox started his professional career as a general pediatrician in 1975, seeing patients in Hays, a town of 18,000 and the major medical center serving a population of 100,000 in the northwest quadrant of Kansas. He arrived with two colleagues with whom he shared a practice and night call. When one partner left, the arrangement became "a setup for burnout." Dr. Cox was also becoming uncomfortable with his skills in the more complex and unusual sorts of cases that occasionally confront a general pediatrician in rural practice.

Then, in the late 1980s he had an epiphany while watching a live newscast from the Gulf War on the evening news. "I could have seen a zit on the correspondent's nose." He reasoned that if television could transmit an image of such high quality from the other side of the world, it certainly could do the same across the state of Kansas.

Bob Cox became possessed that night by the vision of telemedicine he has pursued ever since—one of patients being able to consult with the best doctors for their condition via interactive video. Rural dwellers could now benefit from certain medical expertise heretofore available only by time-consuming travel to urban medical centers. And overworked rural doctors would get some much-needed support in the process.

Dr. Cox immediately began enlisting partners to bring the technical, financial, and organizational expertise he needed to craft a pioneering interactive video system. It consisted of sites at the University of Kansas Medical Center—Kansas City (see "Ace Allen, M.D., pp. 44 and 45), at the University of Kansas Medical Center—Wichita, and at the Area Health Education Center in Hays. The initial plan was to provide expert emergency pediatrics care to patients in Hays by doctors from the big medical centers. The logistics of emergency coverage turned out to be way too difficult. On the other hand, video clinics thrived in pediatric cardiology, neurology, allergy, and psychiatry.

Cox feels that political and economic issues are always bigger barriers to telemedicine use than the technology. He cites lack of Medicare reimbursement as the biggest obstacle today, followed by physician acceptance and bandwidth issues.

Studies have shown the Kansas system, which has spread to all areas of the state since 1991, has been used about 40 percent for education, 40 percent for administration, and 20 percent for clinical purposes. This experience is typical for most interactive video systems and is quite acceptable according to Dr. Cox because educational and organizational support for the practice of medicine in rural areas is every bit as important as direct clinical applications.

For a shy man, Dr. Cox has had to develop a good deal of public speaking skill and political savvy to pursue his dream of connectivity. He left pediatric practice in 1992 to become Medical Director of Rural Development and Telemedicine at Hays Medical Center. He is on the Board of Directors of the American Telemedicine Association, where he has served as Director of the Rural Telemedicine Taskforce. Three of the seven pages of his *curriculum vitae* list presentations done on telemedicine in places ranging from Garden City, Kansas, to Bishkek, Kyrgyzstan and the hearing room of the U.S. Senate Agriculture Committee. "It's clear that almost everything I do is political, carrying a message, influencing."

"We rural practitioners are conditioned to top-down leadership, conditioned to complain when we don't get what we want. We must learn to lead from the community," he believes. "When Hays established its telemedicine connection with the University of Kansas, we found the university lacked rural savvy. When we connected to Ransom, Kansas (pop. about 300), Hays discovered how much it had to learn about frontier medicine."

Dr. Cox currently serves as Medical Director of Hays Medical Center. He is also principal investigator for a Department of Commerce Telemedicine grant for homecare services, the newest installment of the project in Hays. Since his departure from practice, he has helped to recruit thirty new physicians to Hays, including two pediatricians. He believes this success is due in part to the robustness that telemedicine has lent to the Hays medical community. For example, because of its telemedicine program, Dr. Michael DeBakey recently chose Hays as the site for an interactive video presentation on cardiovascular surgery which was broadcast to northwest Kansas and Moscow, Russia.

When asked the secret to his success, Bob Cox says he is a good listener. "I listen to the eyes," a technique perfectly suited to a country doctor who practices telemedicine.

words, painless treatment was not enough to instill full confidence in medical practitioners when death was still a likely outcome of their interventions. Infection claimed just as many lives immediately after the discovery of anesthesia as it had previously.

The second revolution in the modern era of medicine is generally associated with the development of an understanding of the cause of many infections and the corresponding discovery of sanitary practices that prevent the growth of life-threatening bacteria. Many individuals (e.g., Koch, Schwann, Virchow, Semmelweis, and Ehrlich) contributed crucial ideas and observations about the causation of disease throughout the eighteenth and nineteenth centuries, but credit for the revolutionary work is most often given to a French chemist, Louis Pasteur, who conducted a series of convincing experiments in the 1860s and 1870s.

After demonstrating the existence of microorganisms in wine in 1862 and showing how to kill them with heat (the process known ever since as pasteurization), he ultimately turned his attention to bacteria that cause disease and death in humans. Pasteur's work led to the development of the first vaccines during the mid-1880s. Bacteriology quickly developed as a special field of study, producing knowledge of "rational treatment and prevention of infectious disease . . . on an unprecedented scale" by the end of the century.[10]

The hygiene movement also matured during the second half of the nineteenth century. Originally motivated by desires to rid fast-growing cities of stinking garbage and foul-smelling pools of water,

TELEMEDICINE IS . . . RADIOLOGY

For the most part, radiologists are not constrained by appointment time. They are required to be present with patients for a relatively small number of tests (e.g., to inject a contrast medium, to take an image-guided biopsy). Most X rays are taken by radiology technicians, and the developed images are sent to the reading room where radiologists make their diagnoses sitting in front of light boxes hung with films.

Unfortunately, diagnostic images are produced around the clock, and many films arrive at the reading room after the radiologist has gone for the day. The patient's doctor is thus required to do a "first read" and issue a preliminary diagnosis. The radiologist does an "overread" and issues a final diagnosis at a later time—usually after the patient has been treated and sent home. This situation is particularly common in clinics and rural hospitals that are too small to support a full-time staff radiologist. Patients in these settings must often wait for days while the film is sent by mail to a consulting radiologist in another city.

Teleradiology can solve most of these problems. X rays that have been digitized with a scanner-like device or images that were digitally acquired can be sent

sanitation-minded reformers incorporated the concepts of bacteriology into their own work when they learned that epidemics of infectious disease could be traced to grime in the streets. Public health, occupational hygiene, and preventive medicine all developed as respected professions during this *fin-de-siècle* era and provided professional status to the doctors and other health professionals who treated populations and environments rather than individual patients.

Explanations of disease were pure conjecture before Pasteur, but his work created a replicable and explainable foundation for healthcare in the years to follow. Consequently, the revolutionary changes in thought and technology—explaining the origins of diseases and using that knowledge to treat cause rather than symptoms—are commonly categorized as the beginning of the scientific era of medicine. Within just a few decades, medical care moved from a collection of competing and unproven concepts of health to a new model of microscope- and test tube-based medicine. Doctors could now do good rather than just following the ancient dictum to do no harm. The combination of anesthesia and asepsis made surgery safe and effective. Modern medicine now had a foundation on which to build.

REVOLUTION #3: RADIOLOGY AND DIAGNOSTIC IMAGING

Medical care took two great leaps forward with the advent of agents to reduce pain and stem infections, but medical practitioners still had

within minutes over a network (including the Internet) to an on-line radiologist. The radiologist can immediately review the diagnostic studies on a computer screen and return a diagnosis to the treating practitioner, either by E-mail or telephone.

Teleradiology is a win-win technology for all concerned. The image is read by an expert. The referring practitioner and the patient usually won't need to schedule a follow-up visit. Above all, radiologists do not have to run to the hospital at odd hours just to read a single study. They can review images from work stations in their homes, and they can form virtual radiology groups that allow them to provide specialty coverage at any time of day or night.

Radiology was one of the first medical specialties to embrace the technologies of telemedicine, and it will undoubtedly continue to be a leader in the field. National radiology groups are now being formed to give patients and referring practitioners "24 × 7" access to state-of-the-art radiology regardless of location. Price competition can't be far behind.

limited abilities to diagnose many serious problems that might be ben-
eficially treated through an appropriately targeted intervention. With
the exception of externally visible injuries like gunshot wounds and
protruding fractures, tumors and other anatomical anomalies were
still likely to go undetected until irreversible damage was done.

The third revolution in modern medicine occurred with the development of a technology to see inside the body without opening it up
(that is, to explore internal organs noninvasively). Before discovery of
the diagnostic use of X rays in 1895 by Wilhelm Roentgen and similar
developments with radium in 1898 by Marie and Pierre Curie, doctors
could do little more than make educated guesses about the cause of
many illnesses. For example, without risky exploratory surgery, they
could not know with any reasonable degree of certainty whether the
cause of bleeding in a patient's gastrointestinal tract was an ulcer and,
if so, where the ulcer was located. Radiology suddenly helped solve
such problems.

The discovery of the diagnostic power of X rays even had an impact beyond the world of medicine. Conceptual developments in art, literature, and feminism have all been linked to the discovery of this tool
that could reveal secrets previously hidden from view.[11] Ironically, the
rapid expansion of radiology caused many serious health problems in
its early years, before people realized that the indiscriminant use of X
rays could cause debilitating physical abnormalities and death. (The
harmful aspects of ionizing radiation were ultimately harnessed for
beneficial use beginning in the 1930s with the development of radiation therapy to treat cancer.)

X rays brought revolutionary changes to the world of medicine
and launched an ongoing and exciting search for even more ways to explore the body without cutting it open. Computerized tomography
(CT), magnetic resonance imaging (MRI), positron emission tomography (PET), and ultrasound are some recent developments that allow
clinicians to diagnose an ever-growing range of health problems
without resorting to surgery.

This impressive progress is currently marked by the gradual re-
naming of the medical specialty spawned by X rays, radiology. A new
name, diagnostic imaging, is emerging because many of the newer
imaging modalities do not use radiation. Of course, comparable advances in noninvasive diagnostic technology have occurred in other
medical specialties like cardiology (electrocardiography, or EKG, for
studying heart function) and neurology (electroencephalography, or
EEG, for studying brain waves).

The main point for purposes of this book, however, is that radiology represented a revolution in medical practice because it opened

up a whole new realm of possibilities for understanding and treating the illnesses and injuries that require medical care. Noninvasive imaging dramatically reduced the uncertainty that had characterized efforts to understand human health for thousands of years, and it established a new medical specialty that was not dependent on the examination of tissue and fluids. The development of radiology accomplished, within a few years, major and unexpected changes. Telemedicine will be like that, too.

REVOLUTION #4: EDUCATIONAL REFORM

The development of a scientific medical model at the end of the nineteenth century was not immediately translated into uniform, daily practice. Most of the doctors in practice then had been trained before the discoveries of Pasteur and other scientists were incorporated into the medical school curriculum. Their practice patterns were established in the pre-scientific era, when medicine was *only* art.

Even more significantly, the majority of medical schools in the United States did not incorporate the scientific model into their programs after it began to emerge in the 1860s. Johns Hopkins University (Baltimore, Maryland) became the first American medical school to fully embrace the science of medicine when it introduced a new curriculum in 1893 and correspondingly established the M.D. as a four-year undergraduate college degree. Most of the respected state and private universities followed the Johns Hopkins model as they reformed or established their medical schools around the turn of the century, but dozens of other schools continued to graduate large numbers of doctors in much shorter programs that were not fundamentally based in science.

The American medical marketplace in the early years of the twentieth century was correspondingly competitive and chaotic. Doctors not only got little respect, but they also made very little money because there were so many of them. Making house calls and selling various nostrums were necessary to make even a minimal income.[12] Not surprisingly, the university-trained doctors who had spent years learning medicine as art *and* science were bothered by the economic effects of competition from other practitioners who called themselves doctors but did not adhere to the scientific model.

General reform of our nation's economy was occurring at exactly the same time. The Sherman Antitrust Act was passed in 1890 in response to the excesses of monopolies in oil, transportation, and other major sectors of the economy. The Clayton Antitrust Act followed in 1914 to prevent unfair activities that allowed a business to become a monopoly, and the Federal Trade Commission was created in the same year with powers to stop "false, fraudulent, and misleading" trade practices.

The antitrust movement directly addressed the destructive effects of unfettered competition—the heritage of *laissez-faire* concepts advanced by Adam Smith's famous book, *The Wealth of Nations,* published in the same year as our Declaration of Independence (1776). The idea of protecting competition and consumers rather quickly replaced the concept of *caveat emptor* (buyer beware), and government assumed a significant role in regulating economic activity for the first time in American history.

Defenders of scientific medicine were able to benefit almost immediately from this paradigm shift in the nation's economic thinking. With important support from the Carnegie Foundation for the Advancement of Teaching, the American Medical Association's Council on Medical Education engaged Abraham Flexner to visit all the medical schools in the United States. His 1910 report on widespread deficiencies in medical education is probably the best-known of many reform efforts that reinforced the development of state medical practice acts to define the practice of medicine.[13]

Slightly more than a decade later, these educational reforms redefined medical care by limiting the practice of medicine to graduates of university training programs that taught from a science-based curriculum. The adherents of different clinical concepts were effectively

---

TELEMEDICINE IS . . . CONTINUING MEDICAL EDUCATION

Being a good doctor is harder than it used to be. Managed care and tight budgets force doctors to see more patients and do more paperwork, and the knowledge base of medical science is expanding at an unprecedented rate. The net effect of these pressures is that doctors need to know more, but they have less time and money to learn it. The situation is a classic catch-22. Taking time to attend a continuing medical education (CME) program is economically unaffordable, but not taking time is professionally unacceptable.

Through targeted applications of technologies that overcome barriers of time and place, telemedicine is coming to the rescue of beleaguered physicians everywhere. (And we mean *everywhere.* Telemedicine gives equal educational opportunities to doctors in big cities or small towns.) Therefore, web-based continuing medical education will become one of the most successful and visible forms of telemedicine. It simultaneously solves many problems—which is why dozens of course developers and entrepreneurs are scrambling to provide on-line CME.

Of course, home study courses have been available to doctors for many years, but they suffered from many problems: expensive to produce and distribute, quickly

driven out of practice, establishing the medical doctor-controlled model that has prevailed now for almost a century.[14] Ironically, many of the concepts (e.g., herbalism, homeopathy, massage therapies) that were suppressed by Flexner-era reforms are now experiencing a resurgence under the banner of alternative medicine.

Alternative medicine's underworld existence in the United States throughout most of the twentieth century is itself a sign of the revolutionary power of the education reform movement. It defined who was qualified to practice medicine and, in the process of awarding the franchise to scientific medicine, enshrined the role of technology in American healthcare. Above all, the education reform movement reminds us of Victor Hugo's observation, "Nothing is as powerful as an idea whose time has come." Healthcare can be changed, quickly and substantially, by a new idea.

REVOLUTION #5: ANTIBIOTICS AND PREVENTION

The scientific focus of medicine was institutionalized by the beginning of the twentieth century, but the focus of medical care was still treating illnesses that had been the principal causes of death for many centuries. Infectious diseases like smallpox, tuberculosis, diphtheria, tetanus, typhus, dysentery, polio, malaria, influenza, and sexually transmitted diseases were still the primary concerns of medical practice and the leading causes of death.

outdated, presented in a linear format, etc. In contrast, web-based CME can be created with state-of-the-art authoring tools that allow frequent updating and immediate distribution at very low costs. High-quality images and sounds are easily made part of telemedicine CME.

Perhaps most significantly, the nonlinear capabilities of network software allow doctors to gain immediate access to the information they need to learn (e.g., the latest findings about a disease affecting a current patient) and to absorb it at their own speed. Telemedicine CME will also facilitate doctors' efforts to "have a life" because it can be fit flexibly into busy schedules and does not have to be ordered in advance or returned by a certain date.

The number of Web-based CME offerings is expanding rapidly, but interested readers can gain firsthand familiarity with the concept by looking at The Virtual Lecture Hall (http://www.vlh.com), Health Gate (http://www.healthgate.com), and the Medscape CME Center (http://www.medscape.com). To help doctors keep track of all the options, the American Medical Association's CME Locator is an on-line database of over 2,000 available offerings and includes home study courses (http://www.ama-assn.org/imed-sci/cme/cme.htm.)

Hospitals were commonly characterized as places for poor people to die, effectively providing quarantine for poor immigrants who lived in densely populated cities.[15] The wealthy preferred to fight death at home because they perceived correctly that infections proliferated in hospitals. Doctors and nurses treated both groups with care and concern, but they could not do much to change the outcome of infectious disease.

Dramatic progress started to occur in 1929 with Sir Alexander Fleming's chance observation of the bacteria-killing properties of a mold known as penicillin. Research into antibiotics proliferated in laboratories around the world, and antibiotics first became available in general clinical practice during the 1930s. The scientific preparation of vaccinations also prospered, quickly giving doctors the ability to prevent the spread of many of the worst infections. The parallel development of insecticides and pesticides allowed public health officers to make considerable progress against other diseases by eliminating the transmission vectors (i.e., insects and rodents).

The best indicator of the revolution created by antibiotics and related preventive measures is perhaps the redefinition of the hospital. The image of a hospital as "a place for poor people to die" was obsolete by the end of World War II. Beds were no longer filled with people dying from infectious diseases. However, hospital beds were still needed because people were living long enough to develop degenerative diseases. Afflictions such as heart disease, cancer, and stroke became the new focus of medical science and technology.

Replacing one cause of death with another may not seem initially like the result of a successful revolution, but the new diseases did strike their victims much later in life. The relevant point here, however, is that medical care was once again redefined in a relatively short period of time. Doctors and hospital administrators in the 1920s could not have imagined how much healthcare would be changed over the next decade by a chance discovery and the development of science and technology to translate that discovery into daily practice. The medical paradigm had to shift because the underlying circumstances and possibilities changed. By extension, none of us should be surprised that science and technology of the 1990s—in the form of telecommunications and computers—could redefine medicine again within just a few years.

REVOLUTION #6: GENETICS AND PHARMACEUTICALS

The era following the antibiotics revolution may have been one of the longest periods of relative stability in the modern era of American medicine. Most technological advances between the 1950s and the 1980s were refinements of earlier discoveries, and the causes of death remained largely unchanged. The payment system experienced a few mutations along the way, but the day-to-day activities of medical care delivery did not change in any revolutionary way. Practitioners were more preoccupied with battles over "pieces of the pie" (that is, income shares) and specialty turfs than with adopting a new clinical paradigm.

The sixth revolution began rather unexpectedly. The sudden and virulent arrival of acquired immune deficiency syndrome (AIDS) in the early 1980s caught medical science by surprise. Because it was caused by a virus (human immunodeficiency virus, or HIV), AIDS could not be treated with antibiotics. Because it was predominantly associated with sexual behavior, it was politically sensitive. Perhaps worst of all, the replication of the virus defied the prevailing scientific models of reproduction. No one knew what to do to stop the spread of AIDS. The established clinical approaches did not work in treating AIDS, and initial forecasts of its possible progression were quite scary. The word *epidemic* returned to daily use for the first time in several decades.

At approximately the same time, medical researchers made an unrelated discovery about enzymes that dramatically reduced the damage of heart attacks and strokes. First, scientists isolated the tissue plasminogen factor (TPF) that dissolved deadly blood clots associated with both dreaded events. Next, the technologists learned how to grow TPF with an evolving technology based on research with monoclonal antibodies. Finally, practitioners had a new weapon (tissue plasminogen activator, or TPA) to save thousands of patients who would otherwise have died from blood clots in their hearts, lungs, or brains.

The juxtaposition of these two different events may seem odd at first, but they have a revolutionary thread in common. The wars against AIDS and acute myocardial infarction were fought on the battleground of molecular genetics. They are the first highly visible steps toward the widespread, practical application of genetics to medical therapeutics, and they generated incredible interest on Wall Street. Indeed, the investment community became so enamored with the resulting genetics business that hundreds of academic researchers left the security of the ivory tower (i.e., tenure) for the risks and possible rewards of venture capital. Universities began to lose their effective control over the research enterprise, being challenged by the proliferation of for-profit research companies with names like Genentech and Chiron. Commentators began to discuss the arrival of post-academic science.

The most visible evidence of this power shift is probably the human genome project (HGP). Initiated in the old paradigm of government-based research, the HGP is now a race between private and government labs seeking to map the hundreds of thousands of DNA base pairs found in human genes, the first step toward identifying the codes associated with inherited diseases or other genetic abnormalities.[16] Only a few discoveries have been commercialized so far, but the long-run potential for profit is considered enormous.

The successful cloning of mammals in the late 1990s—Dolly, the sheep, being the most famous—raises the possibility of even more therapeutic advances in the near future. "Pharm" animals are already being bred to produce chemicals and tissues that will be among the miracle cures of the early 2000s. In addition, some new drugs are replacing surgery as the therapy of choice for many conditions. Unwanted growths and deposits that were removed by surgeons in the past will be blocked or dissolved by drugs in the future. And biopsies of pathological tissue such as tumors will be cultured in laboratories so that personalized drugs or preventive measures can be concocted on the spot (giving rise to the concept of "designer genes").

Much more can be said about the revolutionary impact of genetics-based pharmacology, but that is not the subject of this book. Our goals in this chapter are to identify new ideas and technologies that have already created discontinuous change in healthcare and to use this knowledge in understanding the implications of telemedicine. The joint development of genetics and pharmacology—like the joint development of telecommunications and computers—is one of those events that is creating a whole new realm of possibilities for healthcare, something much more significant than bringing incremental improvements to the existing system. Although now in its second decade, the pharmacogenetics revolution is far from finished. It will overlap with the development of telemedicine in the coming years. We can all look forward to exciting times in early twenty-first century healthcare as we experience two revolutions at the same time.

THE UNINTENDED CONSEQUENCES OF REVOLUTIONS

Before presenting our in-depth analysis of telemedicine's paradigm-shifting implications in the next chapter, we must make one other point that emerges from the general study of revolutions: in addition to generating many beneficial changes, revolutions also produce problems and surprises. Unintended consequences are part of revolutions. As already shown in Chapter 3, the Industrial Revolution is a good case in point. Its net long-term effects were highly beneficial, but the transition from rural agrarian life to industrialized urban society was accompanied by many unpleasant secondary effects (e.g., smog and teen gangs) along the way.

Unintended consequences are even associated with information technologies that changed the world.[17] Take, for example, the moveable-type printing press. Johannes Gutenberg invented it to spread the word of God by mass-producing Bibles faster than they could be hand-copied by monks. Before long, the printing press was also being used by political and scientific revolutionaries to spread ideas that directly challenged the authority of the church. Alexander Graham Bell developed the telephone to deal with hearing impairment, and inventors of the original computer were only trying to speed up some tedious computations. They had no idea what would ultimately be done with their inventions. They could not have imagined that the telephone and the computer would converge around 2000, enabling the Seventh Revolution in medicine and other remarkable changes.

The six previous revolutions in modern medicine are no exception to the rule of unintended consequences. For example, anesthesia allowed surgery to blossom, but thousands of people died from anesthesia itself before nurses and doctors learned how to manage it properly. Even when anesthesia and surgery were mastered, surgeons performed many operations that replaced one problem with another (e.g., hysterectomies that eliminated fibroid uterus disease but promoted osteoporosis, or prostatectomies that created urinary and sexual dysfunctions in older men who were likely to die of something other than prostate cancer). X rays can both cure and cause cancer, and many "wonder" drugs have been withdrawn from the market upon discovery of deadly side effects. Last, and surely not least, overuse of antibiotics has raised serious concerns about coming epidemics of antibiotic resistant bacteria.[18]

In other words, as enthusiastic as we are about obvious benefits that will come from the telemedicine revolution, we must also recognize the certainty of unexpected consequences. Some unforeseen outcomes will be pleasant, but others will be pesky or even pernicious. The policy analyst's traditional model of cost, access, and quality provides a useful framework for looking beyond the obvious.

> COST: We all know that technology can be expensive. Therefore, in a healthcare system driven in large part by financial imperatives, new technology must be justified economically. One common approach to technology assessment is cost-benefit

PIONEERS IN TELEMEDICINE:
TOM FERGUSON, M.D.

Tom Ferguson, whose on-line E-mail address is at a place called "doctom," says he always wanted to be a doctor. But Dr. Tom is not a guy who examines patients, makes diagnoses, and writes prescriptions. His whole professional career has been devoted to tapping the potential of patients to take care of themselves. He believes that the Internet is the most powerful tool currently available to do just that.

Dr. Ferguson's trajectory in healthcare was set in the late 1960s. As a VISTA volunteer at a migrant program in Florida, he experienced directly how active community participation is crucial to the success of any project. He and his co-workers went to the worker camps, hoping to find sick people who needed healthcare. This approach didn't generate much business in a population that was generally afraid of doctors. When the health workers actually stopped and listened to the inhabitants, they learned that the migrants' biggest concern was inadequate supervision of small children, which had recently resulted in the death of two babies. So the volunteers and residents together developed a daycare center that was a huge, award-winning success.

Later, while majoring in English at San Francisco State University, Tom volunteered at several community clinics, principally the famous Haight-Ashbury Free Clinic. He worked in the laboratory, where one of his jobs was to recruit more lab workers. Inviting patients into the lab to watch their tests being done turned into a successful recruitment strategy. Some people liked what they saw enough to volunteer for training and work. The free clinic movement self-consciously sought to lower barriers between community and professionals—just what the future Dr. Ferguson wanted to see.

After getting a masters degree in creative writing, Tom enrolled at the Yale University School of Medicine, where he edited *Arrhythmia,* the medical student newspaper. His doctoral thesis on the role and potential of self-help and self-care grew into *Medical Self-Care,* a magazine that has reached a circulation of over 125,000. Dr. Ferguson edited the publication for thirteen years.

His full professional life didn't leave room for internship or residency, the graduate medical training he would have needed for a license to practice medicine. Tom says he wasn't interested in practicing medicine within the authoritarian doctor/patient model taught in every training program in the country. Still, he doesn't regret the four years he spent getting an M.D. degree. He feels medical school gave him invaluable insight into

medical language and culture. Tom still reads widely in the medical literature and admits that, "Occasionally, I can even help somebody clinically."

To date, Dr. Ferguson has published thirteen books, on subjects such
as self-care (of course), a medical mystery novel, a children's book complete with stethoscope and, most recently, *Health Online,* a guide to on-
line health information. But today the Internet is the medium for Dr.
Tom. There has been no turning back since he first logged on. The Net is
where he goes to meet most of his own needs for medical information,
where he sends patients and health professionals, and what he writes
and speaks about passionately and prolifically. Tom is credited with
coining the term "consumer health informatics."

Health information is all over the Web. Next to sex, money and E-
mail, health information is the most common use of the Internet. Over
100,000 health-related sites are currently capable of delivering detailed
information on every known medical condition, and the number keeps
growing. Thousands of on-line communities deliver discussion, information, and real support to people with every conceivable medical problem.

Most of this interaction occurs without health professionals. People
seek out the information and contacts that will help them solve their
medical problems. Tom believes health professionals have to accept the
fact that, in this new electronic world, their expertise will be only one
source of information to be tapped and weighed by patients along with
information from medical databases, electronic discussions with other
patients, and alternative medicine resources—all of it laced together
with hot-links.

Savvy medical institutions, doctors, and other providers are getting
themselves into the loop by developing an on-line presence. Helping to
develop medical Internet sites is one of the services Doc Tom provides as
a consultant.

Tom Ferguson's biggest current project is publishing *The Ferguson
Report,* a newsletter about the consumer health informatics industry. It
is targeted to professionals who, like Tom, feel the need to try to keep up
with the fundamental changes that electronics technologies are bringing
to healthcare.

Internet-based information is patient-centered, patient-focused, and
patient-driven. It is just the sort of anti-authoritative model of healthcare
that Tom Ferguson started envisioning in the 1960s. "What's happening is
radical. I don't think that most of medicine has figured it out. I'm just running along behind it, trying to keep up."

analysis. Direct costs—equipment, maintenance, personnel, supplies, and the like—are usually not too hard to determine. Measuring the indirect costs is a bit trickier, and quantifying benefits tends to be even more difficult. How many lives are saved? What about the quality of these lives? Is function improved or, at least, preserved? Should the value of preventive screening be adjusted downward if more information induces misery by worrying otherwise healthy people?

The list of cost-related questions goes on and on, and economists' answers do not always or easily translate into clinically relevant factors like function, longevity, quality of life, or other nonmonetary measures of patient outcome. Political and social imperatives, not to mention lack of valid and reliable data, make economic assessment of medical technology a field fraught with imprecision. Still, our society and political system are demanding more and more economic accountability. Medical economists must respond to this pressure by doing their best to include unintended consequences—both good and bad—in their calculations of the net effect of telemedicine. Otherwise, we will have an incomplete understanding that can lead to poor economic decisions. (Our discussion of the economics of telemedicine in Chapter 7 will reflect an eclectic economic perspective.)

TELEMEDICINE IS . . . PARENTAL BONDING

For the last twenty years or so, medicine has recognized the importance of the relationship that develops between parent and child soon after delivery. Presence of fathers in the delivery suite and infant rooming-in are examples of recent efforts to reinclude parents in the newborn experience.

No matter how great the commitment to keeping baby and parents together, medical complications sometimes require separating them. Technology may often be the culprit that comes between babies and kin (see discussion of fetal monitoring later in this chapter). At least one newborn nursery has used telemedicine technology to bridge that gap.

The University of Tennessee Medical Center in Knoxville (UTMC-K) has a fifty-bed, level-III Neonatal Intensive Care Unit (NICU), able to care for the smallest and sickest newborns from sixteen surrounding rural counties. Occasionally, a baby must be transported to the nursery without the mother, who may be recovering from the delivery in a hospital as far as one hundred miles away. UTMC decided to span that distance electronically. With aid from Ronald McDonald House charities, the

ACCESS: Many Americans are unable to get medical care when
they need it. The barrier attracting the most attention is
insufficient financial resources—that is, having neither
adequate health insurance nor money for out-of-pocket
expenses. Living in a rural area or city center without enough
local health professionals is a close second on the list of reasons
why access is considered to be a serious problem. Of course, we
Americans have never formally committed to healthcare as a
right, but we certainly promulgate a number of policies with the
intent of making sure that everyone has access to healthcare.

The Health Insurance Portability and Accountability Act of 1996
(HIPAA, otherwise known as Kennedy-Kassebaum) is a good example of unintended consequences relative to access. The Act
was supposed to expand the number of people with health insurance (one of its several loosely related goals) by making sure that
employees could change jobs without losing their health plans,
but the number of covered workers has declined by roughly
4 percent since HIPAA's enactment. The Balanced Budget Act
of 1997 (BBA-97) has generated results that are likewise
inconsistent with legislative intent. Medicare+Choice was created to expand options for seniors, but the law's budget cuts actually caused many providers to terminate their participation in
Medicare's new plans. Sadly, legislation to promote telemedicine

hospital installed in the nursery a low-tech, low-cost video system that transmits fifteen to twenty frames per second over regular telephone lines. Three rural hospitals
received complementary systems.

The camera and monitor, mounted on an IV pole that serves as a tripod, are
wheeled to the baby's bassinet in the NICU. At the other end, the mother and family
in the rural hospital watch the baby on a monitor with a set-top camera placed on a
rollabout cart. A telephone closes the audio loop. This is a good time for parents to
discuss their child with a neonatal intensive care unit nurse. Most of the time families just sit there watching their babies.

Observing your newborn child on a television screen may not be nearly as good
as having the baby in your arms. But parents find a video connection goes a long
way towards helping them through the very stressful postpartum period with a sick
baby.

Response to the program has been so positive that UTMC is implementing a similar service, called FamilyTouch, to keep patients from other hospital units in face-
to-face real-time contact with distant family members.

in the future could have the same adverse impact if lawmakers continue to talk one way and then act in another.

Under leadership from the Denver-based Center for the New West, many political and corporate leaders are beginning to address an unintended consequence of the telecommunications revolution—the digital divide created by uneven distribution of high-capacity telephone lines and cables.[19] Unequal access to the Internet could conceivably redefine healthcare's disenfranchised populations by a digital version of redlining. For example, interactive video might bring low-cost home health to a poor person living in a city with a great cable system, while a well-insured patient residing in an area with poor telephone service and no cable might lose access if telemedicine were to replace home nursing services as the standard of care.

QUALITY: Technologies intended to improve the quality of healthcare can be impressive from a purely clinical perspective but counterproductive in human terms. Electronic fetal monitoring (EFM) is an example of how medical technology can interfere with the patient-practitioner relationship and reduce the overall quality of patient care even if it gives more information by tracking fetal heart rate and uterine activity.

Today, on most maternity units, an EFM "test strip" is obtained for at least thirty minutes on every woman in labor, even if she has no risk factors that would suggest the likelihood of fetal distress. If the results are even slightly non-reassuring, the woman will be monitored throughout labor and delivery— meaning that she will be held captive by two large elastic belts which hold finicky monitoring devices against her abdomen. Every time the woman moves, she runs the risk of dislodging one or both of the devices, requiring readjustment by a labor nurse. The fetal monitor machine, often set to make each fetal heartbeat audible on a loudspeaker, stands at the bedside as a constant presence to mother and attendants. Members of the care team may come into her room and look at the monitor strip before they look at her.

This impersonal and "high tech" intervention seems like a small price to pay to reduce the risk of a dead or damaged newborn. Unfortunately, the test is quite imprecise. A questionable EFM pattern is an unreliable indicator of fetal distress, and doctors are frequently faced with the dilemma of what to do about an abnormal result. Often they opt for a cesarean section, forceps, or vacuum extraction. Quite frequently, the baby looks just fine at delivery, showing no signs of the fetal distress indicated by the EFM.

Studies show that fetal monitoring really does give early warnings that save babies' lives when the mother has preexisting risk factors for complications. But studies also indicate that monitoring low-risk labors increases c-section rates without improving fetal outcomes.[20] Nevertheless, electronic fetal monitoring has become a de facto standard for labor and delivery in the United States, a country notorious for its high rate of cesarean deliveries.

In terms of professional liability for acts of malpractice, obstetrics is one of medicine's most risky areas because a "bad baby" (medical slang for an undesirable outcome) can lead to enormous damage awards even when the doctor or nurse midwife did nothing wrong. All other things being equal, a good relationship between practitioner and patient is the best protection against being sued.[21] Still, mainstream obstetrics persists in interposing the fetal monitor between patient and caregivers, even in low-risk patients for whom the technology has been proven to offer no benefit. This practice is emblematic of the broad range of problems that can arise when technology is adopted for technology's sake. It reminds us that the "big picture" can be rather complex, that technology can be a mixed blessing. These cautions should be kept in mind as we now explore the remarkable changes that will be brought about by the Seventh Revolution, telemedicine.

NOTES

1. Webster's Third New International Dictionary (Chicago: Encyclopedia Brittanica/G. & C. Merriam and Co., 1976), 1944

2. Cohen, J. "The March of Paradigms," *Science* 283: 1998–1999 (March 26, 1999).

3. Kuhn, Thomas S. *The Structure of Scientific Revolutions,* 2nd Ed. (Chicago: The University of Chicago Press, Ltd., 1970).

4. Recent events make the authors wonder if anything is permanent in science. Two of the seemingly unshakable certainties of science, the infinite size of the universe and the constancy of the speed of light, are being cast in serious doubt as this book is being written. See Luminet JP, GD Starkman, and JR Weeks "Is Space Finite?" *Scientific American,* (April 1999), 90, and "Slower than a Speeding Bullet" *The Economist* (July 10, 1999), 76.

5. Dyson, FJ. "Miracles of Rare Devices," *The Sciences* (New York Academy of Science, March/April 1999), 32–37.

6. Dyson, FJ. *The Sun, the Genome, and the Internet: Tools of Scientific Revolution* (New York: Oxford University Press, 1999).

7. For further proof of arguments generated by books that categorize significant events in the history of medicine, see the review of Friedman, M and GW Friedland. *Medicine's Ten Great Discoveries* (New Haven: Yale University Press, 1998) in *The Journal of the American Medical Association* 281(15): 1437 (April 21, 1999). According to reviewer Everett Rhodes, MD, "Lists invariably invite seccond-guessing, especially of omissions." His review would suggest that Freud's work and the development of psychotherapy should be included in this list of revolutions. With apologies for excluding psychology and psychiatry from our list of revolutions, we have at least included telepsychiatry and teletherapy as important features of the Seventh Revolution.

8. In order to keep this book readable and on-point, its descriptions of the selected medical revolutions are just long enough to make the key points that help place telemedicine in proper historical perspective. Readers who want to pursue specific knowledge beyond the vignettes presented here will find an excellent summary of the development of modern medicine in Chapters 12–20 of Ackerknecht, EH. *A Short History of Medicine,* Rev. Ed. (Baltimore: Johns Hopkins University Press, 1982).

9. Gauld, A. "Entrancing Influences." *Science,* 283: 493 (January 22, 1999).

10. Ackerknecht, *op. cit.,* 184.

11. Kevles, BH. *Naked to the Bone: Medical Imaging in the 20th Century* (New Brunswick, N.J.: Sloan Technology Series, Rutgers University Press, 1997).

12. The dictionary definition of *nostrum* reinforces the point: "1: a medicine of secret composition recommended by its preparer but usually without scientific proof of its effectiveness 2: a questionable remedy or scheme" *Webster's New Collegiate Dictionary* (Springfield, MA: G & C Merriam, 1980), 778.

13. For a detailed analysis of this fascinating period in the development of medical education and its impact on the subsequent development of healthcare in the United States, see *The Social Transformation of American Medicine* (New York: Basic Books, 1982) by Paul Starr and *American Medicine and the*

Public Interest (New Haven: Yale University Press, 1971) by Rosemary Stevens.

14. The principles of antitrust economics and competition among qualified healthcare practitioners are reexamined in the context of subsequent changes in the education of health professionals in Bauer, J. *Not What the Doctor Ordered: How to End the Medical Monopoly in Pursuit of Managed Care, Rev. Ed.* (Chicago: McGraw-Hill, 1998).

15. For an excellent historical analysis of the development of hospitals, see Rosenberg, CE. *The Care of Strangers: The Rise of America's Hospital System* (New York: Basic Books, 1987).

16. "Big Drug Firms Discuss Linking Up to Pursue Disease-Causing Genes," *The Wall Street Journal* (May 4, 1999), A1.

17. For a detailed and provocative inquiry into unintended consequences in the general context on information technologies, see Levinson, P. *The Soft Edge: A Natural History and Future of the Information Revolution* (London and New York: Routledge, 1997).

18. Garrett, L. *The Coming Plague: Newly Emerging Diseases in a World Out of Balance* (New York: Farrar Strauss & Giroux, 1994).

19. O'Malley, C, R Woodbury, and D Thompson."The digital divide: Small towns that lack high-speed Internet access find it harder to attract new jobs." *Time,* (March 22, 1999).

20. There is a large medical literature to support not monitoring women in labor routinely. Two big studies—MacDonald D, et. al. The Dublin randomized control trial of intrapartum fetal heart rate monitoring. *American Journal of Obstetrics and Gynecology* 152:524–39; (1985) and Leveno KJ, et. al. A prospective comparison of selective and universal electronic fetal monitoring in 34,995 pregnancies. *New England Journal of Medicine* 315:615–619 (1986)—seemed to prove the point definitively. No literature has been published subsequently that disputes the conclusions of the MacDonald and Leveno studies.

21. Levinson W, et al. Physician-patient communication: The relationship with malpractice claims among primary care physicians and surgeons. *Journal of the American Medical Association* 277,7:553–559 (1997).

5

CHAPTER

Telemedicine: Impact of the Seventh Revolution

tele•med•i•cine

 n: combined use of telecommunications and computer technologies to improve the efficiency and effectiveness of health care service; *also* **a** liberating caregivers from traditional constraints of place and time; **b** empowering consumers to make informed choices in a competitive marketplace.

Just as we started Chapter 4 with a traditional definition of revolution from *Webster's Dictionary,* we start this chapter with our own future-oriented definition of telemedicine from Chapter 1. The resulting juxtaposition of meanings is relevant because telemedicine is starting to create a sudden, radical, basic reorientation of our understanding and organization of the healthcare delivery system. Its new tools and paradigms are reshaping the world of medicine as much as the development of a new technology (the telescope) and a new way of thinking (mathematics) allowed Copernicus, Galileo, and Kepler to re-present the solar system in the sixteenth century.

Once again, traditional concepts of space and time will fall. The essence of medical care will no longer be the face-to-face encounter between patient and professional. Thanks to electronic systems, much of medicine will take place without practitioner and patient ever being in the same place or even talking to each other at the same time. For that matter, a lot of healthcare will happen without a doctor or other health professional being involved at all.

Telemedicine will affect every dimension of the relationships between doctors, patients, hospitals, health plans, employers, governments, and other entities involved in healthcare. This chapter considers the evolving impact of telemedicine within the key domains where the effects will be most visible. Our analysis begins with the commodity at the center of this revolution, information itself.

HEALTHCARE INFORMATION

Throughout the twentieth century, healthcare information has existed primarily on paper—textbooks, professional journals, medical records, insurance forms, lab sheets, accreditation reports, compliance studies, legal decisions, strategic plans, etc. Videos and X-ray films are exceptions, but even they have been catalogued, stored, and transported just like paper.

Printed matter has to be physically delivered to anyone needing the information it contains. We have relied on a host of methods—mail, package delivery services, pneumatic tubes, couriers on bicycles—to bring us the desired information in an envelope, box, book, or computer printout.

In other words, the flow of healthcare information in the past was essentially defined by the flow of paper. Much traditional thinking about healthcare and the resulting organization of the delivery system reflects the limitations of the infamous "paper trail." In the future, most health information will flow electronically. We will shift from moving atoms mechanically to moving bits electronically. Moving bits instead of atoms (e.g., paper) is the essence of being digital, in the insightful words of Nicholas Negroponte.[1]

One of the keys to understanding telemedicine's emerging power is to understand the electronic alternative to paper as the medium for storing and moving information. When information is reduced to digital bits, it can move at almost the speed of light, which is considerably faster than the speed of the U.S. Postal Service (derisively called "snail mail" in the wired world) or inter-office couriers. Digital technology also gives us the ability to record information that cannot be stored on paper—information like the actual chest sounds transmitted through a stethoscope, the full three-dimensional image of an ailing brain, or the verbal comments of a paramedic who is so busy saving a life that he or she doesn't have time and a free hand to write them down.

Simply put, digital information can easily be much richer than printed information. Digitization is not just an alternative way to record information that can also be printed on paper; it is also a way to capture additional information. Digitization is, therefore, one of the key advances that makes telemedicine possible and, by extension, will make healthcare different. The databases of twenty-first century healthcare will contain much more than numbers, words, and photographs. They will contain sounds, moving pictures, live sensations, and any other images that can be stored or constructed electronically.

This new and growing scope of information will correspondingly expand the scope of medicine because clinicians will have more ways to record and study what ails us. It will also allow consumers to generate information on their own. Imagine, for example, a homebound patient using a digital camera to take a picture of a postoperative wound or bed sore and downloading the photo directly to the medical record via E-mail. The patient's practitioner then examines this image at a convenient time and place, acts on it, and annotates the picture for the record. Digitization in this illustration produces clinical information in a new way—without the office visit or house call necessary in twentieth century medicine.

However, extending the depth and breadth of healthcare information is probably not the most important implication of digital technologies in general and telemedicine in particular. The big difference is that digital information can be disseminated so easily, which is the reason why telemedicine can be expected to grow so fast.

- Digital information is widely available. It will not be hidden in the closed stacks of academic libraries that seem off-limits to people who don't wear a white lab coat with a stethoscope dangling from the side pocket.
- Digital information is relatively cheap. It doesn't demand the very high prices of medical school textbooks and expensive subscriptions to clinical journals.
- Digital information can be made understandable. With instant links to definitions of key words, explanatory illustrations, and other helpful cross-referenced resources, digital references can pierce the veil of professional jargon that experts often use to obscure simple things.

With such attributes, information technology is a great equalizer, and it is built into almost every form of telemedicine. Digitization and networking will open the knowledge base of health and medical care to anyone who wants to enter it. The twentieth century's medical boundaries—between researchers and practitioners, between specialists and generalists, between physicians and everybody else, between traditional and alternative medicine, between practitioner and patient—will

PIONEERS IN TELEMEDICINE:
DOUGLAS PEREDNIA, M.D.

There may be nothing new under the sun. But the most interesting ideas that arise in our intellectual universe tend to come from new insights that stretch across old disciplines. Douglas Perednia, M.D. got started in telemedicine making one of those multidisciplinary leaps.

As a dermatology resident at the University of Arizona Health Sciences Center in Tucson, he had become interested in dysplastic nevus syndrome, an uncommon skin condition in which the patient may have hundreds of "moles" on the verge of becoming deadly malignant melanomas. The standard procedure is to check each mole every three to six months for evidence of malignant change and remove the ones that appear to be transforming. This is a laborious process in a high-stakes game where error can literally mean death.

Looking for a better way to standardize and document the ever-changing spots on the skin of his patients, Dr. Perednia linked up with astronomers at the Kitts Peak Observatory, located in the desert outside Tucson. Astronomers are passionate about new phenomena that present themselves against the seemingly unchanging celestial backdrop. Nascent blips, representing a host of celestial phenomena from comets to supernovae, contribute crucial data to our understanding of the universe.

Picking out what is changing against a flat, unlit backdrop of thousands of stable celestial objects is a pretty straightforward job, employing computers to compare digitized images captured at two different points in time. When Dr. Perednia attempted to apply the same technology to detecting changes in skin lesions—all the while surviving on "a bunch of $25,000 grants"—he found that job wasn't so easy. Skin must be illuminated. It is three-dimensional and full of hair, pores, and freckles. This dermatologic landscape presents what electronics engineers call a high signal-to-noise ratio. And even with ideally illuminated, color-controlled photos, he found only 85 percent agreement among dermatologists about which lesions were dangerous.

After digitizing the photographs, the next logical step was to transmit them to far-flung dermatologists for their opinions. The images could be stored on computer disks at the receiving site and reviewed at the convenience of the consultants, a classic "store-and-forward" telemedicine application. A number of research papers resulted from these exchanges. Dr. Perednia became a noted authority on the dysplastic nevus syndrome and on how technology might be used to improve managing it, especially for patients who lack easy access to a dermatologist. And, in the case of a relatively uncommon disease such as dysplastic nevus syndrome, the technology could be used to aggregate widely dispersed cases in order to form a sample large enough to generate credible research results.

One of the grants, funded in 1989-90, supported an electronic link between dermatology specialists in Tucson and primary care doctors at an Indian Health Service Facility in Tuba City, Arizona. The project showed that telemedicine could bring specialist services to rural patients. The rural aspect of telemedicine was a natural for Doug. He was raised in Greenville, a "great place to be a kid" small town, midway between Pittsburgh and Erie, Pennsylvania.

As an undergraduate at Swarthmore College Doug majored in economics, which he defines as "the science of making the best of limited resources." This training provided the conceptual base for his involvement in the financial aspects of telemedicine. His first paper, published in 1983, is entitled, "Workplace Fitness with Financial Incentives." Dr. Perednia's writings, speeches, and conversations are suffused with references to the need to justify everything we do in healthcare, including telemedicine, in economic terms. "Telemedicine cannot be something added to the system as an extra cost. It must make people better off, while fitting into the existing cost structure."

After several years of teaching and practice in Tucson, Dr. Perednia moved himself and his family in 1991 to Portland, where he took a position with the Oregon Health Sciences Center. It was a job heavy on telemedicine. He devoted much of his professional life to developing specialty support for the big, largely rural, western state via communications technology. During this time he published a number of seminal papers in the telemedicine literature.

In 1998 he left academia to strike out on his own in the telemedicine field, establishing a consulting business and founding the Association of Telemedicine Service Providers (ATSP), one of the premier organizations serving the telemedicine industry. Not surprisingly, ATSP has a decidedly multidisciplinary focus. Its mission statement includes clinical, economic, political, and educational goals. As such, the industry group reflects its founder, a man whose wide range of perspectives and intellectual honesty have guided and enriched the telemedicine movement. Doug's own words say it best: "Telemedicine has the opportunity to do things right. . . . You can take an area like emergency medicine or dermatology and literally redefine how it is done."

fall as the playing field is leveled by instant, universal access to reliable, well-organized information. (Of course, the elimination of boundaries is not without its dangers. The related pitfalls are discussed in Chapter 7.)

Simplified, expanded, and accelerated access to information not only levels the playing field; it also changes the rules of the game. Physicians have been in control for most of the twentieth century because they knew more than anyone else on the caregiver team. "Doctor knows best," as they used to say, because nobody else had spent so many years learning the facts. But the new information technology means that just about anyone, patients included, can access the same information that is learned in medical school and residency. Key textbooks, refereed journals, up-to-date pharmaceutical references, illustrated anatomical atlases, classroom lectures, diagnostic checklists—all are, or soon will be, on-line and easily accessible.

Open access to the knowledge base changes the skills needed for informed clinical practice. Knowing facts becomes relatively unimportant because computers can store facts better than humans. Knowing how to find and interpret the right information becomes the key to competency. (Besides, the facts are constantly being changed by the cumulative discoveries of the six previous revolutions of modern scientific medicine. The useful life of most medical knowledge is becoming shorter all the time.)

We believe that the implications for physicians are obvious. They must become healthcare's recognized experts in finding and interpreting information, if they hope to take their traditional leadership role into the twenty-first century. They must learn to apply these skills in collaboration with other practitioners and, above all, with patients. In the words of Harlan Cleveland, their challenge is to become *knowledge executives:*

> Every person who seeks or assumes the role of executive leadership in an information-rich society must develop the aptitudes and attitudes of the generalist. . . . The generalist has to be skeptical of inherited assumptions (because some of them are being knocked into a cocked hat by the informaticization of society); curious about science-based technology (because those who would control it must first understand, not how it works, but what it can do for us and to us); broad in their perspective (to take account of the disappearing distinctions between "public" and "private" and between "domestic" and "foreign"); eager to pull people and ideas together (rather than split them apart); really interested in issues of fairness (because the people to be pulled together are); and self-confident enough to work, not in the back room, but riskily out on a limb in our increasingly open society.[2]

We cannot think of any existing group of health professionals more qualified than physicians to become knowledge executives in the new world of telemedicine. We personally know many physicians who are actively and successfully involved in making the shift from selling what they know to working as executives and consultants in the information business. Indeed, most of the innovators behind our "Telemedicine Is. . ." boxes and the "pioneers" in telemedicine (see profiles throughout the book) are physicians. Physicians and other health professionals who accept the implications of telemedicine and embrace the role of knowledge executive will have a bright future. Those who try to defend the old information hierarchy won't fare as well because many consumers will go elsewhere.

TELEMEDICAL RECORDS

The electronic medical record (EMR; also identified as CPR for computerized patient record) has been slowly working its way into everyday use for many years, but generally not as an intentional step toward telemedicine. Most EMR projects have been part of broader efforts at paperwork reduction, including electronic submission of claims (ESC) and electronic data interchange (EDI) projects. The common goal was automation of labor-intensive tasks. Liberating medicine from the constraints of time and place was seldom on the list of objectives, so most of the recent development of EMR should not be confused with telemedicine. (See box at the bottom of pages 92 and 93.)

However, telemedicine definitely benefits from work already done to move medical records from paper folders to electronic files, that is, from atoms to bits. In some enterprise networks, clinicians have been able to access patient records at terminals throughout the health system for several years, and a few such systems have even extended computer links to doctors' offices and homes (especially the homes of radiologists). These early systems fail to deliver on the full promise of telemedicine, however, because practitioners are still tied to a closed network, and patients are excluded altogether.

The revolutionary convergence of technology and thought comes from the idea of using Internet Protocol (IP) to open the records to anyone who can gain access from any location with any available computer. (The security issue is explored in depth in Chapter Seven, where we will show that it is generally blown way out of proportion.) Protected with appropriate access controls, the relevant sections of an IP-enabled medical record can be accessed by any practitioner, not only a family physician at the office but also a consulting clinical pharmacologist taking a break on a ski vacation or a pathologist managing a practice from a home office. We refer to telemedical records to distinguish between this multifaceted, multifunctional record and the plain old EMR.

Of course, for medical records to actualize the full potential of telemedicine, the patient also needs to be in the loop. For example, individuals with chronic conditions can be taught to enter the results of self-administered tests (e.g., glucose, serum cholesterol, functional assessments) directly into their own on-line medical record on a regular basis, thus alleviating the need for an office visit to have the same work done by a doctor or nurse. Implanted or wearable monitoring devices are also being made now with Internet links so that data can be downloaded directly to the medical record on a periodic basis or in response to a crisis. Finally, patients can verbally enter information into their "charts" over the telephone, such as a depressed patient responding to common questions about mental health status.

Telemedical records will quickly become multimedia resources and will include real sights and sounds that are only summarized in words in the paper record, if they are captured at all. Thanks to computers' abilities to search and sort massive amounts of information in just a few seconds, the IP-EMR will also allow specific clinical indicators such as blood pressures or potassium levels that have been collected and filed in different places to be instantly organized in sequence so that changes in a condition can be studied over time.

TELEMEDICINE IS . . . THE PERSONAL ON-LINE MEDICAL RECORD

The medical record is not a top concern of experts preoccupied with cost, quality, and access. Confidentiality is the only related issue that attracts interest, but the medical record merits more attention. Major problems of twentieth century medicine can be traced to this document that is commonly incomplete, out-of-date, undecipherable, and/or unavailable when needed.

The electronic medical record (EMR) is touted as the twenty-first century solution to these problems, but automation alone won't solve them if complete and current information is still not available at the point of service. For example, even if a patient's regular provider has enterprise-wide EMR, no progress has been made if the patient visits an unaffiliated hospital or doctor. The outsiders still cannot access the patient's electronic records because they are not in the same system.

Real progress lies in a complete, integrated, patient-controlled EMR that can be accessed when and where needed. The telemedicine solution is a *network-based* record that is independent of the patient's health plan or provider system. Individuals can compile and store their own medical information at a Website

The telemedical record will further add new dimensions to diagnosis and treatment planning. Because it can be configured to include images taken by a videophone in a patient's home, for example, it will allow clinicians to identify home factors that might contribute to a disease (e.g., a smoking spouse, a filthy deep-pile carpet) or complicate recovery (e.g., several small children who get in the way of adequate rest). Telemedicine allows a clinician to examine his or her patients in their own environments rather than in a medical office—which can dramatically change the evaluative process and improve prescribed therapies.[3]

Last, but not least, the telemedical record expands the possibilities for integrating artificial intelligence (AI) and error reduction into clinical databases. Intelligent agents—sometimes called *bots* to imply a conceptual link to their automated mechanical counterparts, robots—can be used to examine medical information as it flows through networks. These software routines can automatically identify, for example, mismatches between dosage and weight (e.g., an adult-sized pill prescribed for an infant), drug and diagnosis (e.g., a psychotropic medication erroneously being given to treat diabetes), or drug and drug (e.g., incompatible drugs in the same intravenous infusion). As shown by these examples, telemedicine can easily and inexpensively incorporate quality control mechanisms that are simply not part of the traditional paper record. That's revolutionary progress.

---

accessible by authorized caregivers (e.g., participating providers in the patient's health plan) or with special approval given by the individual. This Website can also be a common collecting point for information from many sources (e.g., medical laboratories, diagnostic imaging centers, clinics).

To understand the difference between the old and the new, imagine a man who gets drug prescriptions not only from his health plan's primary care physician, but also from a psychiatrist and another doctor who are outside the plan. He wants an independent clinical pharmacist to review his overall drug regimen, but he does not want his health plan to know about the other doctors. (Admittedly, this scenario is not optimal healthcare, but studies suggest it is extremely common in the real world.) Getting all relevant records to the pharmacist under the old system would be a time-consuming logistical nightmare, if not an impossibility.

Under the new system, the patient will maintain a Net-based record and allow the pharmacist to consult it by providing his personal record access code, just like authorizing a debit card transaction by entering a PIN on a keypad. After the Seventh Revolution, the patient—not the provider—will be able to control the medical record.

RESEARCH

Telemedicine will not only facilitate research by quickly and inexpensively making numbers available for analysis; it will also change the way we look at data to see what makes a difference in the practice of medicine and organization of the delivery system.[4] Research, like the delivery of healthcare it supports, will benefit by being liberated from constraints of place and time.

For example, electronic technology will cause radical changes in the scientific definitions of what "works" in medicine. No longer will the randomized controlled trial (RCT) be the gold standard for establishing medical truth. Rather, solid scientific knowledge will be based upon information systems that constantly evaluate interventions and outcomes in real time. The same data, when batched with financial and managerial information, will allow administrators and systems planners to estimate least-cost combinations of inputs and to allocate resources accordingly.

Research is likely to be changed by telemedicine in several specific areas:

- The information technology behind telemedicine creates the possibility of networked databases encompassing an entire population of comparable patients. Surprisingly, this could mean the end of statistics as we know it. (What a pity!) Conventional statistical analysis was developed in the late nineteenth and early twentieth centuries to permit inferences from small samples to a population because computational methods of the day (e.g., slide rules, paper and pencil) were too cumbersome to evaluate large sets of data. The

---

TELEMEDICINE IS . . . NETWORKED RESEARCH

Everybody in healthcare complains about paperwork. Pharmaceutical and medical device manufacturers probably have reason to complain loudest. For the best of motives—to protect the public—the Federal Food and Drug Administration requires extensive studies and reams of reporting on every new drug and medical device before it is allowed on the market. The requisite investigations demonstrating safety and efficacy can cost hundreds of millions of dollars. A fair share of those millions is spent on paperwork.

Phase Forward, a Waltham, Massachusetts firm, created InForm, an integrated system for collecting and monitoring clinical trial data. Because it is Web-based, InForm software can receive data from multiple sites and forward it to a central

technologies underlying telemedicine will allow nearly instantaneous computations with massive data sets, so inference—with all its limitations and its requirement of random selection—will not be necessary in many situations. The vexing problem of how to compare information from small sample sizes will also disappear in the process.

• The new databases that can be constructed from telemedicine's distributed networks will dramatically reduce the time needed to analyze data and translate new knowledge into daily practice. For example, due to methodological requirements of RCTs for most of the twentieth century, conclusions could not be drawn until sampling data had been analyzed at the end of an experiment or other research study, causing a typical study to last three to five years from start to finish. The time and money costs of sampling commonly prohibited interim analysis, too. Now, with data collection from entire populations occurring over the Internet just as soon as information is recorded, data can be analyzed at any time. The databases of telemedicine will also begin to overcome one of the major limitations of RCTs, namely, the lack of information about treatment effects in the years *between* the beginning and end of an experiment.

• The overall quality of research should improve because standardized data collection methods can be built into the computerized interfaces between clinicians and patients. Telecomputing as a research tool should eliminate some of the bias that compromises many studies, such as strengthening the "double blind" mechanism used to insulate researchers and

database at the moment it is entered. The electronic database gives authorized project personnel instant access to up-to-the-minute information, no matter where they are located and what time they log-in.

InForm services start at $50,000 to support a single trial of limited size. The folks at Phase Forward believe that the time and resources saved by automating data collection, collation, and reporting make InForm a bargain. And, if it lives up to its promise to shorten time to market for new products, the savings on paper goods will just be gravy. Effective drugs and medical devices will get to market much faster.

For a firsthand view of this new approach to data collection and research, visit http://www.phaseforward.com.

subjects from knowing whether a treatment is the experimental effect or the placebo.[5] Research protocols can be embedded in the data collection process at all times, incorporating AI routines for early identification of the flaws that have invalidated many a study in the past because problems with the data were not discovered until the end of the experiment. Even longstanding problems with inter-rater reliability—the degree of consistency *between* different observers making subjective judgments about clinically relevant changes—should be improved by telemedicine's multimedia capabilities. Researchers can use calibrated scientific instruments (e.g., densitometer, colorimeter) to make side-by-side comparisons of actual pictures in telemedical records, a highly desirable alternative to the longstanding practice of basing comparisons on numerical rating scales or verbal descriptions.

- Telemedicine has the potential to reinforce experimental controls, the steps intentionally taken to insulate an experimental effect from other factors that might explain variation in observed outcomes at the end of the study. The issues of compliance and persistence, for example, are good cases in point. Results of drug studies are occasionally cast in doubt by the possibility that patients in one of the groups might not have filled their prescriptions (compliance) or taken the prescribed drug as directed for the entire course of treatment (persistence). Telemedicine can address the problem by capturing data from pharmacies' prescription records, and research subjects can be required to report taking their pills through an on-line reporting system. (Increasingly, patients are being paid to participate fully in medical research, so getting them to provide information may become less of a problem than it once was.) Measurement error is another research problem that can be addressed by telemedicine. For example, on-line data collection instruments can include standardized scales and conversion tables to reduce measurement error that is commonly introduced when patients respond to open-ended questions or fill in blanks on written forms. Electronic responses can also be monitored continually, allowing researchers to find and fix items that elicit inconsistent or meaningless responses.

These illustrations of telemedicine's potential advantages are incomplete with respect to the future because they are presented in the context of traditional approaches to research. Looking ahead, we see that modern information technology creates opportunities to investigate massive amounts of data in ways that could not have been imagined as the RCT was refined over the past century.

The future databases of telemedicine are particularly ripe for a relatively new form of analysis called data mining. Its methodologies are still being developed, and its results certainly do not meet scientific requirements for demonstrating causality.[6] Associational at best, the results of data mining can nevertheless yield useful and valuable information. Marketing applications of this new tool are already helping firms in other industries (e.g., banking, entertainment, insurance) to identify the characteristics of good customers and to target promotional campaigns accordingly.

> As companies collect more information about customers, they see patterns emerging. Wal-Mart Stores Inc. has used data collection to formulate "market baskets" of typical shopping trips. Reebok's. . . Internet site allows companies to track how customers scrutinize a product, down to fabric preference. An Internet site lets companies watch how customers focus on various features of products, and they can see when people buy, and when they just browse and leave.[7]

Parallel applications in healthcare are not hard to imagine. Health systems will surely start digging into telemedicine's databases for similar marketing purposes, particularly as the medical sector becomes more competitive.

This brief introduction to key issues barely scratches the surface of the many ways in which telemedicine will change and improve research. (For a specific example, see "Telemedicine is . . . networked research" on pages 94 and 95.) Other dramatic changes will undoubtedly emerge as clinical researchers and computer scientists develop closer working relationships, and we are confident that bigger and better databases will be among the most enduring contributions of the Seventh Revolution.

HEALTH INSURANCE

Linking health insurance to telemedicine may seem like a stretch at first because potential relationships between the two topics have received little or no attention to date. However, we believe that significant changes in reimbursement will be promoted by the merger of telecommunications and computers. Stated conversely, some much-needed improvements in third-party payment would be unlikely to occur without telemedicine, but they will happen sooner or later because the telemedicine revolution is already underway.

PIONEERS IN TELEMEDICINE:
RON POROPATICH, M.D.

Ronald K. Poropatich coaches his son's soccer team, first because he is intensely dedicated to his children and second, because keeping up with a gang of ten-year-olds helps him stay in shape for skiing. On the slopes, he likes to go "deep and steep." In fact, a review of his professional and personal accomplishments suggests that his approach to every experience is to go deep and steep.

Dr. Poropatich chose his medical specialty, pulmonary critical care, because of the depth of its challenges. Dr. Poropatich explains that taking care of the sickest patients demands a breadth of medical knowledge that constantly tests his limits. Rising to a challenge also explains why he has succeeded so well in the world of telemedicine.

When Ron is not addressed as "Dr. Poropatich," he is likely to be called "Lieutenant Colonel Poropatich." He joined the Army Reserve Officers' Training Corps as an undergraduate studying biochemistry at the University of Pittsburgh. Then, while on active duty, he earned a masters degree in microbiology when he wasn't "jumping out of airplanes and helicopters."

Laboratory work at Walter Reed Army Medical Center brought him in contact with the medical world. Ron set his sights on medical school. He attended Hahnemann University in Philadelphia and returned to Walter Reed for seven years of internship, residency, and fellowship training. He stayed on there to serve as director both of the medical intensive care unit on the pulmonary critical care service and of the tuberculosis program.

This combination of assignments may have been a full life for most people, but Dr. Poropatich was looking for something more. In 1991, at the height of the conflict with Serbia, this son of two Croatians volunteered to use his vacation time to do humanitarian work in Croatia. The Army vetoed that idea, so in 1992 he volunteered to go to Kenya to minister to Somalians fleeing their country's civil war. Again, the Army said "no go."

In late 1992, when the United Nations assembled a peacekeeping force in Somalia, the U.S. military remembered Ron Poropatich from his previous attempts to volunteer. They chose him to lead the telemedicine charge into that African nation. Ron knew next to nothing about telemedicine, a new set of technologies that the downsizing military had been developing to support its medical mission worldwide. Within three weeks, Dr. Poropatich was on a C-5 transport aircraft headed to Somalia. He carried a Macintosh portable computer which would be a critical component of the system used to relay medical data from forward positions back to support doctors as far away as the United States.

In 1995 he became director of the Telemedicine Directorate at Walter Reed and was also made responsible for networking telemedicine care delivery in the twenty-one-state region served by Walter Reed. Thanks to his involvement with telemedicine, Dr. Poropatich has since been deployed in Hungary, Kenya, Croatia, South Korea, Haiti, Macedonia, and Argentina. He has also been to the White House and discussed telemedicine with the President and Vice President. "It's been an incredible adventure," he says.

In 1997 Dr. Poropatich added to his portfolio the directorship of the Clinical Applications Division of the Telemedicine and Advanced Technology Research Center (TATRC—see Chapter 6 and References). His job is to coordinate development and installation of telemedicine systems within the military. Some of these systems sound like devices out of science fiction. For example, a new miniaturized transducer applied to the scalp uses sound waves to measure the stiffness of the skull. It gauges pressure inside the head, data previously available only in the intensive care unit with an instrument inserted through a hole in the bone. Now, critical data on head-injured soldiers can be acquired and transmitted from the front lines to clinical experts at distant military hospitals. "Acoustic hemostasis," using high-intensity focused ultrasound waves to stop internal bleeding without breaching the skin, is another of the amazing technologies on TATRC's horizon.

As far as telemedicine is concerned, Poropatich feels that "these are the good old days." Increasingly sophisticated technology is coupled with administrative and financial support of a mission that the military deems critical to its ability to sustain troops and civilians, in peacetime and at war. Thus far, the estimated military investment in telemedicine is approaching $350 million, with no sign of diminishing.

Dr. Poropatich is aware of the constant need to justify technology in terms of cost, access, and quality. Early results are very promising. Active military programs in dermatology, dentistry, child psychiatry, nutrition, and echo-cardiography, to name a few, are proving the potential of telemedicine. Extensive distance education offerings in healthcare add further value.

In his experience, freedom from civilian constraints, such as cross-state licensing and reimbursement, plus a disciplined environment make the military an ideal place to pioneer some of these technologies. While practicing, teaching, and publishing in his medical subspecialty, Dr. Poropatich continues doing a couple of full-time jobs promoting telemedicine in the military. "We're still on the steep part of the learning curve," says Ron Poropatich. Fortunately, being in steep situations is just where he seems most comfortable.

The reimbursement process is heavily automated, but it still involves an incredible amount of paperwork and human intervention. (See the box at the bottom of the page.) Therefore, telemedicine is likely to change the health insurance business because it solves so many problems associated with paperwork handled by humans. For example, identical copies of telemedical records can be sent to multiple sites in seconds at almost no marginal cost, ending one of the biggest bottlenecks in the payment process.

The claims review process can already be facilitated by—and maybe someday replaced with—intelligent agents (bots) and other AI applications. Digital pictures embedded in the patient record will allow reviewers to see injuries, surgical repairs, functional impairments, and other clinical details that often become the subject of prolonged dispute and delayed payment. Verification of eligibility and benefits is currently being accomplished over the Internet in real-time (that is, no waiting). And once new security systems such as retinal identification and electronic fingerprinting are fully integrated into networks, telemedicine will be a highly effective weapon in the fight against insurance fraud.

Telemedicine will even improve actuarial analysis because insurance carriers will be able to use researchers' data collection tools (see previous section) for focused studies of special populations. The speedy ability to assemble databases for population-based studies should someday soon promote price competition between insurance companies because groups or individuals seeking a bid can make their utilization data available with relative ease.[8]

The historically significant price advantage for group health policies should even decline or disappear altogether because an IP-based

---

TELEMEDICINE IS . . . HEALTH PLAN BENEFITS VERIFICATION

Almost anyone with health insurance has firsthand experience with the hassles of verifying benefits at a doctor's office, hospital, pharmacy, or other care delivery site. Finding covered services and participating providers or verifying deductibles and coinsurance payments has often turned a short visit into a long one. Even worse, preliminary eligibility determination at the point of service can be followed by a particularly unpleasant surprise—the retroactive denial—when health plans announce that benefits were changed just before the encounter.

Printed benefit materials simply cannot keep up with the changes inherent in today's topsy-turvy world of managed care. Only the health plans' computers can stay current, which creates many delays and other problems when doctors' offices and hospitals are forced to rely on outdated directories or patients' old insurance cards because they are not tied to the fiscal intermediary's computer.

computer system can process thousands of individual policies as easily as it handles the transactions for one group plan with thousands of members. The payment mechanisms of E-commerce will soon be developed to the point that collecting premiums from individuals will cost very little more than getting one check from a corporation.

Telemedicine's power to reduce administrative barriers between patients, providers, purchasers, and plans should soon reinforce growing efforts to shift the control of health insurance from employers to individuals. As reflected in a recent statement by the president of the American Medical Association, more and more people are coming to the conclusion that meaningful health reform will not be possible in the United States as long as health insurance is a benefit of employment:

> Let individuals select and own their own health plan. It just makes good sense to put decisions about health care directly in the hands of those receiving the care.[9]

Dr. Dickey's concept of transferring health plan control from employers to individuals with a corresponding shift from defined benefits to defined contributions will be much easier with the help of telemedicine than without it, particularly because telemedicine's most revolutionary effect is likely to be patient and consumer empowerment (see final sections of this chapter).

The next logical step is development of radically different ways to buy and sell health insurance, and we don't need to look any further than the securities business to see what could happen. Thanks to the same types of computer systems that have revolutionized stock transactions, we can hazard an intelligent guess that individuals in 2010 will be buying highly customized health plans with premiums

Beginning in early 1999, Blue Shield of California started to allow physicians to have direct access to computerized membership eligibility information via its corporate Website. Participating doctors and their office staff can now connect directly with www.blueshieldca.com to verify eligibility and benefits and to get other important information like drug formularies and Blue Shield's policies and procedures. The site also allows members to verify status of an existing claim and review an explanation of benefits statement. (See McCormack, J. "Why Build an Interactive Site?" *Health Data Management* (March 1999): 78.)

Telemedicine will reduce uncertainty in the realm of reimbursement as its technologies enable an increasing number of on-line linkages between health plans, providers, practitioners, patients, and purchasers. The various parties will not necessarily be happy with the correct information they retrieve through on-line inquiries, but at least they'll know the situation.

based on individual experience and health profiles—all via the Internet. For example, a single airline captain in her forties might solicit several on-line bids for a plan with no maternity benefit, first-dollar coverage for cancer and heart problems, catastrophic coverage for all other conditions, a national practitioner panel, and a wellness incentive rider.

Maybe this scenario sounds too far-fetched. But would you have believed us back in 1990 if we had predicted that you would be able to manage your own investment account and do your own securities trading by the end of the 1990s? Would you have listened when we warned you not to buy stock in the big-name, old-line brokerage firms that used to manage your portfolio because many of them would disappear? Well, both happened.

So, don't be too surprised if today's on-line stock brokers are among the many different businesses competing for your health insurance dollar ten years from now. Computers and telecommunications have redefined the formerly staid worlds of investments and banking in less than a decade. What's to prevent a similar transformation on the financial side of healthcare?

DELIVERY SYSTEM

Our healthcare delivery system has been characterized over the past few decades by an increasing concentration of self-contained business entities. Hospitals have been the predominant economic unit, and sectoral growth has been accomplished primarily through mergers and acquisitions of existing hospitals ever since the Hill–Burton program stopped providing easy start-up capital in the 1970s.[10] Consolidation, much of it with money from for-profit corporations, occurred at a rapid pace throughout the 1980s. Hospitals grew into vertically integrated health systems by purchasing collaborators all along the supply chain (e.g., medical groups, freestanding emergency centers, outpatient surgery facilities, nursing homes and retirement communities, etc.). Physician practice management (PPM) companies and a few other horizontally focused firms tried to carve out specialty niches, but none has transformed the industry as originally promised or feared, and some have gone bankrupt.

Much of the concentration of ownership might not have occurred if industry leaders had foreseen the coming development of telemedicine. The consolidation binge reflected an industry-wide assumption that health systems had to own the locations where scheduled medical services were delivered. Indeed, before the telemedicine revolution, owning clinical outlets "all over town" was arguably a good competitive strategy because providers needed to offer convenience; that is, to minimize customers' travel time to a system-owned location that could meet their needs.

Now, along comes telemedicine with technologies that virtually redefine the places and times of customer-provider interaction. Health systems should ponder lessons that can be learned from the computer industry which has already been changed dramatically by an upstart, Michael Dell, who turned lack of ownership of a conventional distribution outlet into a strong competitive advantage.

> . . . Dell has bypassed traditional distribution channels and gone directly to customers. Most important, perhaps like Amazon.com Inc., Cisco Systems Inc., and a few other companies, Dell helped pioneer the almost end-to-end use of digital networks to communicate with its customer, take orders, and then pull together products from suppliers.[11]

As noted at the beginning of the referenced article, astute application of telecomputing technologies has already created a new word, "*delled* —to be outflanked by cheaper products from a thoroughly digitized Dell." We will not be at all surprised if health care executives in the early years of the twenty-first century talk about being *kooped* because they quickly lost so much business to a former U.S. Surgeon General who digitized basic health services, completely bypassing ownership of hospitals and other traditional delivery settings.

If you do not understand or accept the possibility of being kooped, you need to spend a few hours visiting drkoop.com and similar Web sites that are identified in Chapter 8, Annotated References. You won't have to look too far below the surface of these sites to see how several well-financed visionaries are creating telemedicine-based networks. These sites will compete directly with local health systems that continued to invest heavily in bricks and mortar when they should have been spending some of their money on electronic infrastructures. Healthcare's longstanding "edifice complex" is becoming counterproductive.

The future belongs to delivery systems with good portals to the Internet and superb abilities to focus clinical resources in a variety of new ways. Physical presence will be an issue, but the keys to success will be different. In some situations, central supply warehouses and package delivery services (e.g., contracts with FedEx or UPS) may be the best way to meet customers' needs in their homes and places of employment. Drive-up kiosks may become the specimen collection centers of the future. Mobile clinics and testing centers may also play a role. The point is that telemedicine will change customers' expectations.

Capital investments should be made to optimize customer service in a medical marketplace very different from the one we have known for the last forty to fifty years.

The old goal of owning and controlling the entire healthcare delivery chain (i.e., vertical integration) is not the wave of the future. Rather, the telemedicine revolution will likely establish virtual providers—relatively small, entrepreneurial management organizations that assemble an integrated delivery system from disparate sources—as the predominant type of healthcare organization over the next decade. Therefore, progressive health systems must immediately start thinking and acting like general contractors, creating electronic networks of qualified subcontractors that can be instantly integrated upon demand to provide top-quality medical services in virtual time and space.

PRESCRIPTION PHARMACEUTICALS

The pharmaceutical industry may be the bellwether for the future of healthcare. It is a driving force behind the pharmacogenetic revolution (#6) as shown in Chapter 4, and major drug manufacturers are making significant investments in information infrastructure.[12] Pharmaceutical companies have acquired some of the nation's largest networks of medical information (e.g., MerckMedco, McKesson/HBOC) over the

---

TELEMEDICINE IS . . . ON-LINE PRACTICE MANAGEMENT

Practice management tasks have been automated, but not integrated, for several decades. A doctor's office might use one software package for financial management, a different vendor's product for tracking clinical information, a hospital's scheduling system, and so on. In addition, doctors are starting to use E-mail to communicate with hospitals, colleagues, and patients.

Each automated function is helpful by itself, but overall results fall far short of potential in the absence of integration. Money is wasted when medical offices pay for several systems that don't work together. Major savings and operational improvements can be achieved by bringing all management functions together in a single, open-system network. Inter-office linkages are becoming important, too, as managed care creates incentives to form "medical groups without walls."

Physician practice management (PPM) companies dazzled Wall Street in the mid-'90s when they captured impressive front-end profits by integrating practice management within and between the medical practices they acquired. PPMs then crashed in 1998 because they underestimated the difficulty of managing diverse physician groups. Telemedicine creates big opportunities for companies that can

past few years and now own comprehensive data on virtually every aspect of the healthcare business. Clinical pharmacists with doctoral degrees (Pharm.D.) are quietly mastering the skills of information management, with excellent potential to rival physicians as knowledge executives in the new world of twenty-first century healthcare.[13]

With all these changes and with drugs replacing surgery as the therapy of choice for a growing number of medical conditions, the pharmaceutical sector will likely become even stronger in the coming years. Spending on prescription drugs has consistently hovered around ten cents on the healthcare dollar for the past several decades, but the sector's relative share of all medical expenditures has recently started to rise and is likely to continue growing for the foreseeable future. (Therefore, expect the issue of Medicare drug benefits to move into center ring of the Washington health policy circus.)

Unlike some prominent hospital systems and healthcare management companies, pharmaceutical companies have positioned themselves well for the sixth and seventh revolutions through investments in information and related partnerships. The pharmaceutical sector has also started to learn how to conduct business electronically. New on-line pharmacies, such as planetrx.com and drugstore.com, are attracting considerable attention at the end of the decade. An initial review of healthcare's answer to amazon.com suggests that the first electronic drugstores need to work on a few rough edges, but they offer

provide physicians with integrated practice management services without forcing them to abandon their independence.

To see how doctors will use communications technology and computers to achieve efficient practice management without selling their practices and their souls, visit WebMD (http://www.webmd.com). One of the first companies to provide doctors with single-source, on-line practice management, WebMD already bundles key functions into its subscription service, including real-time verification of insurance coverage, telephone triage through a single number, professionally staffed on-call answering service, customized Website support, and direct links to basic references (e.g., medical libraries, drug information, and interactive anatomical charts).

WebMD has arranged strategic partnerships with direct links for subscribers to buy medical supplies, books, insurance, transcription services, mortgages, and investments. WebMD is also positioning itself to serve as an interface (maybe even matchmaker?) between physicians and patients by establishing a parallel Website for consumers. It also merged with Healtheon and formed partnerships with Microsoft, Intel, and Superior Consultant (among others) in early 1999. As they say on the evening news, stay tuned for further developments in this fast-breaking story....

great promise—especially in contrast to national chain drugstores with "long lines, poorly informed help, impersonal service, and confusing organization of the merchandise."[14]

With the arrival of on-line pharmacies, patients do not need to take paper prescriptions to the corner drugstore because clinicians can submit them electronically. (Of course, the clinician-patient encounter that generated the prescription could also occur on-line.) Patients can use E-mail to ask a pharmacists about their prescriptions or check the site's database for possible side effects and interactions of the drugs they are taking. The on-line pharmacists can reply not only with answers to each patient's questions, but also with related attachments and hot-links that promote understanding of the diagnosis, the prescribed therapy, and preventive self-care. The prescribed drug is then sent to the patient by mail or package service, with express delivery options if time is of the essence.

The on-line pharmacy is pure telemedicine in the making. It will ultimately be much more efficient than the way Americans have been filling their prescriptions for the past hundred years, and it clearly liberates caregivers and empowers consumers. Sure, we'll continue to grouse about the loss of "mom and pop" drugstores on main street, but we've been lamenting their disappearance for the past twenty years and still switched our business to Wal-Mart or the Rite-Aid by the mall. Will we now feel sorry for the retail chain stores as they experience on-line competition? Probably not. . . telemedicine is different.

PATIENT-PRACTITIONER RELATIONSHIP

Electronic technology will unquestionably enhance our power to heal. It will even supplant the need for human interaction in treating many conditions. Telemedicine is already reducing the need for healer and patient to be in the same place at the same time, but for the foreseeable future—the authors' forecasting horizon on this point is a decade or two ahead—no technologic advance will replace the practitioner-patient relationship. Change it, yes, but not replace it.

We have intentionally chosen a comprehensive term, *practitioner-patient relationship,* as a substitute for the traditional reference to *doctor-patient relationship.* Nonphysician practitioners such as physician assistants, nurse practitioners, certified nurse-midwives, nurse anesthetists, clinical psychologists, and physical therapists ably deliver a large amount of healthcare that is wholly compatible with the reigning paradigm of allopathic medicine. And as already noted in a different context, much has been made of traditional medicine's recent "discovery" of the enormous amount of care provided by naturopaths, massage therapists, herbalists, shamans, and other practitioners from outside the scientific ranks.[15] Because we believe that telemedicine will expand the range of health practitioners even further, eventually blurring distinctions between traditional and nontraditional, we have chosen to use "practitioner" throughout this book (except in direct references to physicians) because of its inclusiveness.

Practitioner is not a perfect solution, however, because it still sounds a bit too unidirectional for our tastes. It doesn't reflect the growing importance of two-way exchange, a central feature of communications in the electronic age. Bidirectional (or even multidirectional) interchange between patient(s) and healer(s) is a critical human factor in telemedicine. For lack of a better word, *practitioner* and *practitioner-patient* will have to suffice, but readers should keep in mind our belief in the power of a meaningful two-way or multidimensional relationship where each party brings valuable information and worthy feelings to the exchange.

The practitioner-patient relationship has been at the center of healthcare since the beginning of time. Every culture or belief system has caregivers whose job is to be the conduit between the patient and the healing force. Whether that force is rooted in modern science or possessed by Mother Earth, God, the gods, stars, or a human deity doesn't matter. The intercessor, whether doctor or shaman, must relate to both the patient and the greater universe. This relationship is healing itself.

Plenty of scientific evidence in the standard medical literature supports the healing powers of the relationship,[16] and anybody whose career is devoted to caring for patients will tell you the same thing. We consequently believe that both patient and practitioner will need to learn how the healing relationship is affected by telemedicine. For example, many patients will enjoy their newfound electronic ability to gather and evaluate lots of information before interacting with a practitioner, but others will still expect the doctor to know best. Some people will likely put more trust in the results of their Web searches than in the counsel of experienced practitioners. On the other hand, a few will undoubtedly collect massive amounts of information—much of it unfocused or irrelevant—and then expect the doctor to review it all and decide what to do in the old autocratic manner.

The point is that telemedicine will probably create all sorts of new patient types, which by extension will create a variety of relationships with practitioners. Practitioners will need to be prepared to deal with patients who have different amounts of information and attitudes about how it ought to be reflected in clinical encounters. Diversification of relationships is the most likely result, so any discussion of telemedicine's impact on *the* patient-practioner relationship would be a misleading oversimplification.

Indeed, a practitioner's policy for dealing with information provided by patients may become an important differentiating factor in an increasingly competitive market. It will also become a significant consideration in professional liability (an issue discussed in depth from the perspective of public policy in Chapter 7). Years of experience have shown that misunderstandings and other human problems in the patient-practitioner relationship—not deficient care—are the main reasons for malpractice litigation, so practitioners will have good reason to think defensively about their on-line presence.[17]

Telemedicine also means that the best experts will be orders of magnitude more available to patients. Geographical barriers, which have been toppling since the Industrial Revolution, will continue to fall. Both sides of the relationship can benefit from the development of national markets for health services. Within a decade or two, patients will be able to "shop" for practitioners who offer the desired mix of specialized competence, information, and care. Specialists will be able to be correspondingly selective, using electronic tools to channel specific patients into their practices.

TELEMEDICINE IS . . . VIRTUAL HOUSE CALLS

The house call is one of our country's most cherished memories of medicine back in the "good old days." Indeed, the home visit by a doctor may be the enduring emblem of the golden age of American medicine. It disappeared when doctors became dependent on hospital-based technology and when insurance companies—not patients—started paying most of the bill.

House calls may have yielded to efficiency and technology, but some clinically important benefits were lost in the process. The home visit gave doctors an opportunity to evaluate patients' surroundings, seeing firsthand factors that might explain illness or delay recovery. It also allowed the patient to stay in a familiar setting, avoiding the stresses and exposures that accompany visits to a clinic. House calls contributed to curing and caring, as well, because the doctor could teach the rest of the family what to expect and how to help. For lots of medical problems, there is no place like home.

Telemedicine now makes possible the twenty-first century equivalent of the home visit—the virtual house call. Inexpensive devices can be placed in the home to monitor vital functions twenty-four hours a day and give immediate warnings when

Paradoxically, telemedicine will allow care to be more individualized as the underlying technology becomes more general. Herein lies the great potential of new technologies to bind patient to practitioner. The transition from the traditional relationship to many new ones will not always be smooth, and it won't happen overnight. But telemedicine will make sure that it happens.

SELF-CARE AND HOME HEALTH

In the process of liberating medical care from longstanding constraints of time and place, telemedicine will allow some untraditional settings to blossom as care sites. More medical services will undoubtedly be delivered in schools, workplaces, and commercial locations (as shown in several "Telemedicine is . . ." boxes), but the greatest area of growth will probably be self-care in the home. (See the box at the bottom of the page.) People will have unprecedented opportunities to get the care they need without leaving their place of residence.

For example, many will benefit from the rapidly advancing technology that is bringing interactive video into the home at a reasonable cost. Currently, the quality of video is reduced when it is transmitted over regular telephone lines. The screen image is relatively small (compared to the full-screen size of commercial television), and motion looks

---

signs point in a bad direction. An interactive video link can be established between home and clinic—allowing *prn* (as needed) face-to-face interactions between patient and practitioner. A distant health professional can electronically watch the patient take a pill, examine the patient's body for bed sores, even make sure the refrigerator and pantry contain foods that will promote recovery.

Unlike early (i.e., mid-'90s and before) telemedicine interactions that required patient and caregiver at prescheduled times to go to mini-studios with bulky equipment linked by costly cables, the new telemedicine is made possible by small and inexpensive devices that can be hooked up to a regular residential telephone. The cost of an integrated home monitoring unit is now less than $500 and falling.

Today's telephone-based virtual house calls will be replaced more and more by television visits—which explains why telcos have been busy buying cable companies in the late 1990s. You may soon have the opportunity to be the first person on your block to see your doctor between sitcom reruns, all without leaving the recliner in front of the home entertainment center. Ma Bell will become Doc Bell, figuratively speaking. Whether the fee for the visit will be included in your monthly cable bill is an open question.

PIONEERS IN TELEMEDICINE: DENA PUSKIN, Sc.D.

The government could not have found a more dedicated or qualified expert to serve as Director of the Office for the Advancement of Telehealth (OAT) when OAT was established in early 1998. Dena Puskin was present at the beginning of the federal government's renewed interest in telemedicine during the late 1980s. No other civil servant has done more or started earlier to promote technologies that overcome time and distance barriers to healthcare.

While studying for a doctorate at Boston University in the late 1960s, Dena became involved in community action activities, which ultimately led her to leave laboratory science for a career focused on overcoming barriers to healthcare. Her social concerns resulted in terminating her research on the biochemistry of hemoglobin to take a job with the New York State Health Department and help create a healthcareers recruitment and training initiative for the Rochester area.

After creating the initiative, she was selected as the first full-time student in a new master's degree program in community medicine at the University of Rochester, where she learned how to get things done within the establishment and work creatively within a bureaucracy. Having established her credentials in health services research, she was recruited into the doctoral program at Johns Hopkins University. Her graduate advisors included many of the country's most respected health policy experts of the 1970s and beyond (e.g., Drs. Kerr White, Salkever, Starfield, and Horn). Her work with Kerr White focused on the extent of primary care services provided by medical specialists, an issue still debated today.

Upon completing her dissertation, Dr. Puskin returned to Rochester to work on cost-containment policy as the Director of Research and Evaluation at the Finger Lakes Health Systems Agency. She was responsible for overseeing a wide range of research and evaluation activities, including the development of budget models to allocate resources from the perspective of the entire community rather than competing hospitals. Dr. Puskin also taught epidemiology at the University of Rochester School of Medicine.

Upon leaving the Health Systems Agency in 1981, Dr. Puskin joined the Rochester Area Hospital Corporation, a community agency that controlled the allocation of hospital revenues in Rochester. While developing quantitative methodologies to support collaboration among hospitals, she became very interested in the relationships between technology and access. She dedicated considerable effort to identifying money wasted in duplication of technology and finding ways to redirect it to services that would improve the community's overall welfare.

Dr. Puskin moved to Washington, D.C. when her husband took a position with the Nuclear Regulatory Commission. She began her Washington career in the legislative division of the Blue Cross and Blue Shield Association, where she became involved in national health policy issues such as tax caps, healthcare vouchers, and state rate setting. She also helped prepare the Blues for their role as intermediary under the new Medicare Prospective Payment System (PPS).

When the Prospective Payment Advisory Commission (ProPAC) was created to advise on the implementation of PPS, Dr. Puskin returned to government service as one of ProPAC's first policy analysts. She was primarily responsible for developing the initial economic framework to update PPS payments (including those to adjust for technological developments), and examining rural payment policies. When Congress created the federal Office of Rural Health Policy (ORHP) in the late 1980s, Dr. Puskin was the obvious choice to serve as its Deputy Director.

Within two weeks of joining ORHP, she was asked to oversee a major telemedicine project in West Texas. The rest, as they say, is history. Her successful management of multiple-agency funding for this demonstration project was followed in 1994 by creation of the Rural Telemedicine Grant Program that has supported over 400 telemedicine facilities in forty-four states. She is an advisor on telemedicine policy and program development to a large number of organizations, including the Healthcare Financing Administration, Department of Defense, the Federal Communications Commission, the Senate/House Ad Hoc Committee on Telemedicine, and the White House. She has been chair of the federal Joint Working Group on Telemedicine, the interagency group that coordinates programs and policies across federal agencies, since its founding in 1995.

Her credentials as a pioneer in telemedicine are first rate, but she modestly shares the success with others. "The telehealth movement is about creating new opportunities to improve healthcare and get services to people who would otherwise be outside the system, but no one can do it alone," she says. Dr. Puskin gives special praise to her staffs at ORHP and OAT and to the grant recipients who have worked together to develop telemedicine programs cooperatively rather than competitively. Her many collaborators return the compliments and note that no civil servant has done more to advance telemedicine. If federal leadership in telemedicine might be characterized as a team activity, Dena Puskin deserves special recognition as a visionary and dedicated coach.

jerky because the frame rate is usually reduced (from thirty frames per second for full-motion video to less than fifteen frames per second for video transmitted over telephone line). Fortunately, the future looks better, both literally and figuratively.

Dramatic advances in compression technology are enhancing the quality of signals sent over regular telephone lines, but the future lies with cable in most markets and with satellite links in others. AT&T's acquisition of MediaOne and TCI in 1999 is perhaps the most visible example of cable's future role in putting all forms of communication, including telephone and Internet, on cable. Home health will be an obvious beneficiary because millions of residences are already hooked up to cable, and cable has the bandwidth to support sophisticated telemedicine. Hundreds of new ventures will take advantage of the situation, and much healthcare will be delivered in the home, soon.

Portability and miniaturization of Internet-enabled monitoring equipment also allows practitioners to follow more patients where they live. Fewer patients will need to leave home for lab tests, for example, because the necessary equipment can be brought into the home and monitored over telephone lines or cable. Visiting nurses or therapists can also make periodic visits and bring along specialized equipment that is too technical or too expensive to leave in the home for the duration of an illness or injury.

Last, but not least, patients will have access to an incredible amount of on-line support to help them take care of themselves. The Internet provides access to thousands of Web pages with multimedia information about condition-specific advice and treatment options. On-line support groups are proliferating at an incredible rate.[18] Again, a few growing pains are to be expected as telemedicine brings more healthcare directly into the home, but long-run advantages greatly outweigh the short-term problems. In the future, telemedicine—not a daily apple—will keep the doctor away. (Of course, doctors who haven't adapted to the changes will complain a lot and may even be reduced to selling apples.)

EMPOWERED CONSUMERS: CLINICAL PERSPECTIVES

The preceding sections of this chapter have shown many ways in which the healthcare game is a lot more complex than it used to be. Competition is becoming more intense now that data travel almost anywhere in the world at the speed of light on the command of a few keystrokes, and hoarding information no longer confers any significant strategic advantage. Because everybody has more information—and increasingly the same information—interpreting it well and applying it wisely become the new keys to success. (Ironically, misinformation may become a powerful weapon in the future, but that's another story.[19])

Electronic communications media have opened the universe of healthcare studies and opinions to laypersons via radio, television, and now, computer. Physicians learned a long time ago to watch "60 Minutes" and listen to National Public Radio in order to obtain some advance warning of the medical news stories that their educated, middle-class patients would be asking them about. In the last few years, the number of electronic sources of medical news has grown explosively, ranging from consumer-targeted television ads for prescription drugs to thousands of medically-oriented Websites and talk shows hosted by all manner of doctors and other healers.

Practitioners in every field are finding that their patients are better informed (or, at least, more informed) than they used to be. Patients ask more questions. They routinely do research about side effects of drugs before having prescriptions filled. And every day more patients are quoting to their doctors information they have found on the Internet.[20] The patients of at least one practicing physician (Ringel) are even starting to bring lots of downloaded printouts to appointments and to E-mail pertinent Web sites. Discussions with other practitioners suggest this phenomenon is now rather common. Thanks to widespread exposure given to medical topics by the media, a constantly growing number of patients expect their practitioners to know what's happening on medicine's leading edge.

What does this mean to the health professional? It means that the balance of power has shifted. Professionals derive their power in large part from their monopoly on the body of information that their specialty controls. In modern times, the patient-doctor relationship has hardly been between equals. Doctors know a lot more about medicine than patients do. To put information in the hands of patients— especially if that information is reliable and well organized (not at all to be presupposed in today's information anarchy)—is to put more power in the hands of those patients.

With the help of electronic media, patients can now shop around for healthcare, and they can do it without making and keeping appointments at inconvenient times. They have access to information about institutions, about pharmacies, about physicians, about other practitioners of traditional medicine, about providers of alternative medicine, about self-care, healing communities, and so on. Patients are becoming empowered consumers, turning providers and practitioners into vendors who must please their customers in order to survive.

Access to information is causing dislocations all over the medical food chain. Patients are not the only ones who have found new muscles to flex. Generalists (such as family doctors, general internists, and pediatricians) have seen their credibility, value, and even their incomes increase as subspecialists lose their grip on the unique information that defined their domains. Non-physician practitioners such as nurse-practitioners, physician assistants, and nurse midwives, are moving into some of the niches previously reserved exclusively for physicians. No group of health professionals can control information technology or telemedicine.

On the other side of the practitioner-patient relationship, an increasingly powerful consumer will bring many changes to the whole system of medical care.

- Empowered patients will expect individualized care. As shown in Chapter 3, the transition from industrial society to information society means that goods and services, including healthcare, will be targeted to smaller and smaller groups of consumers. Thanks to telemedicine, patients will be better able to make sure the care they get is the care they want.

- Empowered patients will dictate the quality of care they desire. Informed patients will drive the system with their own expectations about the appropriateness and safety of the services they receive. They will be able to compare practitioners, health systems, and health plans because they will have a variety of on-line databases to access for information on quality.

- Empowered patients will embrace location-independent care. They will not be forced to go to a doctor's office or a hospital for many services because the care will be available electronically in a variety of convenient settings. If the need arises to consult the world's greatest expert on a particular problem, telemedicine will make it possible even if the specialist lives half-way around the world.

- Empowered patients will impose globalized standards. Telemedicine will mean the end of the community standard for medical care. National practice standards, based on the best available data, will become the norm. No longer will practitioners be able to defend themselves against malpractice claims by asserting that they were adhering to the local way of doing things.

As shown by these examples, empowered patients and their advocates will more than ever be in the position to insist on the services that best meet their individual needs. In turn, providers of clinical care will need to be attuned to consumers' clinical expectations because "shopping around" will be so easy in the world of telemedicine. If patients don't like the care they are getting from one provider, they will be able to go somewhere else without leaving home. Of course, costs will also be a consideration, so we'll conclude our analysis of the telemedicine revolution with a review of its economics.

EMPOWERED CONSUMERS: ECONOMIC PERSPECTIVES

The empowering force of telemedicine is being concentrated and accelerated by a much larger, even global, revolution with significant economic dimensions far beyond health care. Its enabling technologies are giving consumers new power in many areas of their daily lives, as indicated in comments by Steve Case, the CEO of America Online (AOL):

> " . . .the Internet empowers people in ways that were not possible with television or newspapers. With these broadcast-type media there was a producer or an editor making decisions for the audience—deciding what they should see or hear. That simplified things, and it also deprived the audience of the full range of choices."[21]

To see how these media-focused comments relate just as well to telemedicine, substitute "post-World War II healthcare" for "television and newspapers" and "a doctor or an insurance company" for "a producer or an editor." With these changes, healthcare consumers are definitely part of the "audience" deprived of the full range of choices.

For this reason, Case's general point about information-based consumer empowerment applies to health care at the beginning of the twenty-first century. Doctors and insurance companies have controlled more than the clinical decisions about our health care. Ever since payment for medical services shifted from predominantly out-of-pocket to predominantly third-party, doctors and insurers have also controlled our consumption via the "power of the purse."

Once veterans' organizations and labor unions enshrined health insurance as a basic benefit during the 1950s, American consumers quickly fell into the trap of buying their healthcare on the basis of what doctors and insurance companies would allow. The idea of consumers spending their own money to get the health services they want was lost. Most health economists—the present one (Bauer) among the exceptions—therefore assumed that consumers did not shop for medical care because purchasing decisions were made on their behalf by doctors and insurance companies. As a reflection of this assumption, most textbooks on medical economics prominently include a "healthcare is different" statement within the first few pages.

One reason for this assumption is consumer ignorance, a rather inelegant term of economic art. According to the theory of consumer ignorance as applied to healthcare, patients can't know enough about health and illness to make intelligent decisions. Only the doctor possesses the knowledge to make the right diagnosis and select the appropriate therapy. In other words, only a doctor is qualified to decide how a patient's insurance resources should be allocated.

Consumer ignorance is not the only way in which "healthcare is different" in the eyes of a typical economist. Since the 1960s, mainstream microeconomic analysis of medical markets has also been based on the concept of market failure, the idea that classic laws of supply and demand do not apply to healthcare because patients do not have to pay for their care. Health economists have assumed for years that 80% of all healthcare spending is controlled by the producer (doctor), not the consumer (patient).[22] More recently, a comparable proportion of physicians believes that the power to make medical decisions has shifted to the Health Care Financing Administration (HCFA) and managed care organizations (MCOs).

The practitioner-payor debate over who should control health care consumption is raging at the turn of the millennium, but the adversaries seem to have missed the importance of another shift in economic power that is taking place at the same time—specifically, the resurgence in consumer payment for healthcare. Quietly, relentlessly, and without meaningful political debate over its desirability, consumers are paying more and more of the total healthcare bill. (Control over health plans and payment for medical services are two different

---

TELEMEDICINE IS . . . INFORMED PATIENTS

Information is power. Health information has the power to heal—especially in the hands of those who need it most, the sick. For the CHESS program, developed at the University of Wisconsin, patient empowerment is the primary goal.

"CHESS" stands for "Comprehensive Health Enhancement Support Systems." It is a Web-based service designed to help patients with serious illness—including breast cancer and HIV infection—to cope at home. A modem-equipped personal computer provides access to medical information, personal stories, support services, medical experts, and to other patients with the same disease. CHESS even includes software-based routines that, for example, lead a woman through a branching decision tree that helps her decide if she should have a simple lumpectomy or radical mastectomy for her breast cancer.

Initially developed for use by more educated patients, CHESS has been tested in multiple populations, including impoverished inner-city African-Americans.

issues. In an ideal world, individuals would control their health plans, and employers and governments would pay the premium. Unfortunately, this isn't an ideal world.)

The important point for our purposes here is not that most medical economists were wrong in the past. Rather, we believe they are short-sighted if they continue to accept the conventional wisdom that consumers are not significantly involved in the payment for health services and don't know enough to make intelligent decisions. Economists and other policy analysts need to change their way of thinking because the underlying circumstances are changing. In fact, any historical justification for assuming market failure in health care is rapidly eroding as responsibility for payment is shifted back to patients (where it was before the 1950s):

- Personal experience shows us that health plan deductibles have risen from $100—the norm throughout the 1980s—to amounts five to ten times higher by the end of the 1990s.

- Over the same period, we have seen co-insurance rise from the long-standing rate of 20% to rates as high as 50% for out-of-plan coverage under many managed care plans.

- The proportion of health maintenance organizations charging a copayment of $10 or more per physician visit rose from 34% in 1993 to 70% in 1997.[23]

- The employee share of the premium for single coverage increased 284% between 1988 and 1996, but the employer contribution rose only 79%.[24]

Wherever it has been installed, CHESS has been extensively used and highly praised by patients. Studies have consistently found that users have a higher quality of life while consuming fewer medical resources than patients with the same disease at the same stage who lack access to the system.

People with severe chronic disease are at risk for isolation brought on by the disabilities that accompany their affliction. One study found that AIDS patients used CHESS on average 138 times for 39 hours of on-line interaction in the course of three to six months. The connection to professionals and compatriots had become a critical part of their support system in the face of a relentless disease.

The CHESS system has also been adapted to support heart disease patients, students in academic crisis, families of substance abusers, caregivers of people with Alzheimer's disease, and victims of sexual assault. The model appears to have endless potential because it is based in a source with endless potential—the people themselves—and allows them to use it in a convenient, unscheduled time and place.

- The medical savings account (MSA) option under Medicare+Choice includes incentives to return unspent health dollars directly to patients.
- According to state regulators, individuals' premiums are climbing at least twice as much as the increases in group policy premiums that employers face in 1999.[25]
- Consumers are already spending as much of their own money on alternative healthcare (estimated at $27 billion) as they are spending on all outpatient physician services.[26]

The last item on this list is especially important because it contradicts the common assumption that people won't pay for their healthcare. (The vexing problem of people who can't pay for their care is addressed in Chapter 7.) The staggering out-of-pocket amount paid to alternative practitioners should disabuse anyone of the notion that consumers have become totally dependent on third-party payment. More than it would like to admit, the mainstream medical community is already engaged in a major economic battle with sellers of alternative services. Traditional providers ignore the significance of self-payment at their own peril, particularly if the competition harnesses telemedicine more quickly or effectively than they do. Telemedicine will quickly become a major weapon in the economic battle for out-of-pocket dollars, and nothing can be done to keep telemedicine out of the competition's hands.

From the perspective of economic theory, telemedicine will also expand the market through a price effect—the part of the law of supply and demand that says consumers buy more when prices fall. Telemedicine will ultimately make healthcare less expensive and more cost-effective (as argued in Chapter 7), reinforcing consumers' willingness to purchase more healthcare and spend more of their own money on it. Depending on the price-elasticity of demand for medical services under these new circumstances—an important but unknown factor at present—total spending on healthcare would not necessarily rise even though people were buying more of it.[27]

All the changes discussed in this chapter point toward a medical marketplace very different from the one Americans have known since health insurance took hold after World War II. Individuals are regaining control over their health plans, employers and governments are quietly shifting payment responsibility back to patients, consumers are starting to spend more of their own money on health services, and as much as half of those out-of-pocket dollars are being spent on alternative services.

At the very same time, telemedicine is providing patients with unprecedented access to clinical information, as shown in the previous section. A growing number of consumers are comfortable using the tools of telemedicine to gather and evaluate information that was previously controlled by doctors. Not too far into the first decade of the new millennium, the parallel trends in payment and information will have reinforced each other and created a truly competitive market for medical services.

Individually controlled health plans and informed consumer choice—not market failure and consumer ignorance—will be the prevailing economic features of the new medical market. Medical economists will be totally absorbed in trying to understand the competitive dynamics of a "level playing field" where supply and demand really work. Their belief that "healthcare is different" will become part of twentieth century economic history. By empowering consumers, telemedicine will make sure that the health economy works like markets for other goods and services.

COMPLETING THE METAPHOR: WHAT GOES AROUND. . .

We began this chapter with a brief historical reference to Copernicus, Galileo, and Kepler. Their use of two new tools, the telescope and mathematics, produced not only a jarringly different world view, but also one with enormous power to predict the movement of heavenly bodies. These early scientists demonstrated that the earth rotated around the sun, not vice versa.

Life quickly became uncomfortable for religious leaders and kings whose authority derived from self-proclaimed links to the higher authority that had presumably created the earth at the center of the universe. Established rulers tried hard to suppress the new paradigm, but they failed. They fell victim to an uncontrollable flow of information propogated by a new medium—books printed on a moveable-type press.

The metaphorical value of the sixteenth century revolution in cosmology should not be lost on any healthcare professionals who believe the world of healthcare revolves around them. Hospitals and doctors *were* at the center of the twentieth century medical universe. They could expect consumers to come to them because that was the way the system worked. The masses didn't have a vision of anything different.

But once again, fundamental relationships are being rearranged by a new flow of information and a different world view. Telemedicine will put consumers at the center of the healthcare universe in the early decades of the twenty-first century. Providers will revolve around the consumer, not vice versa. And as historian George Santayana has so perceptively noted, those who do not understand the lessons of history are doomed to repeat it.

NOTES

1. Negroponte, N. *being digital* (New York: Alfred A. Knopf, 1995).
2. Cleveland, H. *The Knowledge Executive: Leadership in an Information Society* (New York: E.P. Dutton, 1985), 5.
3. The authors thank Jay Sanders, M.D. for private communications with specific examples to support this point.
4. For a comprehensive and comprehensible introduction to the fundamental concepts of statistical analysis, see Bauer J. *Statistical Analysis for Decision-Makers in Health Care: Understanding and Evaluating Information in a Competitive Market* (Chicago: McGraw-Hill, 1996). This unconventional statistics book anticipated the changes that medical informatics and telemedicine are bringing to research in healthcare, so it will be useful to readers who want to understand theoretical issues surrounding new techniques for data collection and research method.
5. "Double blind" refers to the concept that neither patients nor researchers know who is getting the actual treatment and who is getting the placebo treatment; that is, they are both "blinded." By comparing the experimental group, which got the treatment being studied, to a closely matched control group, which got the sham treatment, double blind clinical experiments are meant to eliminate the bias of patient and researcher expectations from their conclusions.
6. The scientific concept of causality was originally elaborated by eighteenth century philosophers like Isaac Newton and Francis Bacon. It sets forth rigorous criteria, such as covariation (that is, where one quantity changes, the other changes with it), that must be met before one event can be said to cause another.
7. Wysocki Jr., B. "Corporate Caveat: Dell or Be Delled," *The Wall Street Journal* (May 10, 1999), A1.
8. This possibility may renew the public policy debate over experience rating versus community rating in health insurance. Proponents of both positions will likely have better data to defend their positions, but the outcome of the debate will depend at least as much on political conditions at the time.
9. Dickey, NW. *American Medical News* (November 16, 1998).

10. The federal Hill-Burton program was established in 1946 to provide generous matching grants to communities that wanted to create more hospital beds. Thousands of new or expanded community (that is, not-for-profit) health facilities were constructed throughout the entire country with Hill-Burton funds, particularly in the 1950s and 1960s. However, the program was curtailed in the early 1970s when policymakers became concerned about an oversupply of hospital beds. The rise of private, for-profit funding in the hospital sector during the 1980s is arguably a result of the disappearance of the federal money. Investment capital had to come from somewhere since Hill-Burton hospitals were beginning to show their age, and Wall Street was attracted by the profit potential in healthcare.

11. Wysocki Jr., B. op. cit., A1

12. For an in-depth analysis of the pharmaceutical industry, its applications of information technology, and its relationships with other key sectors of the medical economy, see Bauer, J. "The Changing Paradigm of Knowledge in Health Care: Implications of Evolutionary Experience in the United States," in *Proceedings of the High-Level Seminar on Production, Mediation, and Use of Knowledge in the Health and Education Sectors,* (Paris, France: Organization of Economic Cooperation and Development, 1999).

13. A detailed review of pharmacists' expanding roles is presented in Chapter 7 of Bauer, J. *Not What the Doctor Ordered: How to End the Medical Monopoly in Pursuit of Managed Care,* op. cit., 147–155.

14. Mossberg, WS. "Online Drugstores Offer Some Remedies and a Few Headaches" *The Wall Street Journal* (April 29, 1999), B1.

15. The seminal article that forced contemporary American medicine to recognize the pervasiveness of nontraditional practices was Eisenberg, DM, et al. Unconventional medicine in the United States. *New England Journal of Medicine.* 1993;328,4:246–252. Further substantial growth in use of non-traditional medical resources was documented in Eisenberg DM, et al. Trends in alternative medicine use in the United States, 1990–1997. *New England Journal of Medicine* 289(18):1569–1575, 1998.

16. See, for example, *Healing Words* by Larry Dossey (HarperCollins, New York: 1993).

17. See, for example, Levinson, W et al. "Physician-Patient Communications," *Journal of the American Medical Association* 277(7): 553–559.

18. "Patient Forums: Self-Help Medicine" *Medicine on the Net* (May 1999): 7–13.

19. According to J.R. Wilson, military strategists are devoting considerable resources to the dissemination of false information and other forms of information warfare (which has already earned its own acronym, IW). See his article, "A New Kind of Warfare," in *MIT* 3(1): 32–34. (www.MIT-kmi.com)

20. Data available in the late spring of 1999 suggest that anywhere from 30 to 60 percent of all Internet users have sought health information at some time during the past year. The data are inherently imprecise because use of on-line resources is growing exponentially. However, the rate of growth is effectively the point. The number of people using the Internet for health information is already large and growing fast. Those who doubt the staying power of this phenomenon should ponder the comments of David D. Alger, CEO of a prominent New York-based investment firm. "I am often asked: how many of those Internet companies will survive? What we should ask is: how many of their non-Internet-based competitors will survive?" *The Wall Street Journal* (April 26, 1999): A18.

21. Although perfectly relevant to this discussion of consumer empowerment in health care, Mr. Case's comments were made in response to inquiries about the Internet's role in the tragedy at Columbine High School in Littleton, Colorado. They are included in Thomas L. Friedman's Foreign Affairs column, "Judgement Not Included," that appeared on the editorial page of *The New York Times* (April 27, 1999): A31. The title and concluding sentence of Mr. Friedman's editorial launch an important issue that we will revisit with respect to healthcare in later chapters: "The more the Internet makes us all broadcasters, all researchers, all consumers, and alas, all potential bomb makers, the more critical it is that our teachers, parents, and communities are still making us all citizens."

22. This figure, 80 percent, appears so commonly in medical economists' studies that it has gained respectability through repetition rather than research. The authors are not aware of a body of published literature that has consistently demonstrated an effect of this (or any) magnitude. The actual percentage of consumer spending controlled by physicians is unknown and probably unknowable, but it has surely been substantial for the past several decades.

23. HCFA, Office of the Actuary, *Health Affairs* Nov–Dec 1998.

24. Lewin Group, Inc., quoted in *USA TODAY,* October 23, 1998.

25. *The New York Times,* December 5, 1998.

26. Eisenberg, DM et al "Trends in Alternative Medicine Use in the United States, 1990–1997" *Journal of the American Medical Association* 280, (18):1569–1575 (November 11, 1998).

27. Price-elasticity of demand is a measure of the relative change in quantity demanded associated with a relative change in price. Total spending (price times quantity) is a direct function of elasticity. If total health spending does rise as a result of telemedicine's price effect—something that would concern policy-makers who still have a twentieth century view of the world—consumer welfare may actually increase because the market will presumably be more competitive, that is, consumers will have made the decision free of anti-competitive constraints. However, the theoretical details are beyond the scope of this book, and any effort to apply them here would be highly speculative since medical economists know next to nothing about the price-elasticity of demand for healthcare in competitive markets. Interested readers can learn more from any basic textbook on microeconomic theory, and all readers should appreciate the fact that this discussion was relegated to an endnote.

6

CHAPTER

Trends in the Technology of Telemedicine

The history of telemedicine directly reflects the development of enabling technologies, so a focused discussion of technological trends is now needed to complement the review of telemedicine's revolutionary impact (Chapter 5) before the overall analysis can be completed in consideration of policy issues (Chapter 7). In the process of laying foundations for the future, this chapter demonstrates the powerful momentum behind technological developments that will free healthcare from the limits of space and time and empower its consumers.

Technology is commonly defined as the application of science to practical purposes. Unfortunately, the typical dictionary definition of *technology* does not even hint at the dizzying rate of change that can be experienced in specific applications like telemedicine. We know that many aspects of our discussion will be quickly outdated by new discoveries and unexpected developments, so we have prepared a section of annotated references (Chapter 8) to be used as an aide for keeping track of subsequent change.

Of course, key scientific and technological terms are used throughout this chapter. Basic explanations are provided in the text, and more-detailed and cross-referenced definitions are provided in the glossary (Chapter 9). With all these tools, readers should be prepared to become active participants in the Seventh Revolution because the enabling technologies are rapidly becoming user-friendly, affordable, and accessible.

FEDERAL LEADERSHIP IN TECHNOLOGY DEVELOPMENT

People who like to criticize the federal government should think twice before discrediting its role in the research and development of telemedicine. Sure, bad law and inept bureaucracy have a way of creating some pretty big messes in healthcare, but telemedicine is not one of them. The development of telemedicine as science applied to practical purposes is arguably an example of government doing something right and—for the most part—doing it very well. It is also a good example of sound public investment with returns to the private sector for benefit of the general welfare. To give credit where credit is due, the U.S. federal government deserves recognition for exemplary leadership in the technological aspects of telemedicine. (We carefully distinguish technology from policy. As we will show in Chapter 7, Medicare reimbursement for telemedicine is anything but progressive.)

The story begins approximately forty years ago when the National Aeronautics and Space Administration (NASA) first faced the challenge of providing health services to astronauts. Although the initial, short-duration missions did not require overcoming the barrier of time, they most definitely confronted the barrier of space—outer space. NASA's medical scientists and engineers had to develop many new ways to monitor health signs at a considerable distance, so some of the earliest work in telemedicine was a direct result of the "space race."

In need of remote sites to test systems being developed by Lockheed, NASA collaborated with the Indian Health Service (IHS), the branch of the Public Health Service (PHS) responsible for providing care to Native Americans. Medical support links were established between NASA facilities and the Papago Indian Reservation in southern Arizona, creating Space Technology Applied to Rural Papago Advanced Health Care (STARPAHC). The government effectively got two benefits for the price of one project: technology development for the space program and healthcare for a remote, underserved population. NASA continues to be heavily involved in telemedicine, including projects to develop portable instrumentation packs and to improve satellite transmissions of medical information.

The next large federal program addressed the special needs of a new medical school serving roughly 40 percent of the state of Texas. This sparsely populated area presented special challenges for health educators who were supposed to train students throughout this massive service area, so an interactive video system was installed with a major grant from the U.S. Public Health Service. The project, started in 1989 and called HealthNet, linked faculty in the four medical campuses of Texas Tech Health Sciences Center and provided a productive environment for early development of video consultations, continuing education via satellite, and diagnosis over telephone hookups (e.g., radiology, pathology, monitoring).

Several other federal agencies also became involved in supporting technological developments in telemedicine at approximately the same time.[1] The Rural Utilities Service, a branch of the Department of Agriculture, began to operate the Distance Learning and Telemedicine (DLT) Program under the 1990 Farm Bill. It has awarded many grants to rural schools and healthcare providers for investments in telecommunications systems and equipment. The Indian Health Service has continued to expand its activities beyond STARPAHC, and the National Institutes of Health's National Library of Medicine (NLM) has supported the development of telecommunications infrastructure that meets the information needs of clinical care and research. Within the Department of Veterans Affairs, the Veterans Health Administration (VHA) has developed many networks to support healthcare for veterans at hundreds of V.A. medical centers and clinics around the country.

Rural health has probably been the most visible area of federal involvement in developing technological infrastructures for telemedicine. Several hundred grants to rural health providers have been made since 1994 through the Rural Telemedicine Grant Program and the Rural Health Services Outreach Program. Initially administered by the Office of Rural Health Policy (ORHP) to address rural health needs, program management was transferred in 1998 to the newly created Office for the Advancement of Telehealth (OAT), which focuses on the needs of all medically underserved areas.

These program activities tended to emphasize applications of interactive video. They did not generally attempt to develop new technology, focusing instead on finding ways to use commercial, off-the-shelf (COTS) interactive video systems for clinical care, administrative functions, and professional education. Although the rigidities of multi-year grants effectively prevented grantees from adopting newer technologies as telemedicine evolved beyond interactive video, the recipients of federal funds became a close-knit group and shared their experiences at regular meetings around the country. Several of today's leaders in the telemedicine industry emerged from this network.

The grant-funded projects included evaluation components to provide information about costs and benefits of different approaches and the extent to which objectives were met. The data from many of these evaluations are being used by the Health Care Financing Administration (HCFA) to establish federal policy for reimbursing telemedicine, a problem addressed in the next chapter.

DEPARTMENT OF DEFENSE

Since necessity is aptly characterized as the mother of invention, we should not be surprised that the most creative leadership in telemedicine technology came from the armed forces. While civilian agencies were largely exploring interactive video as a new solution to an old problem—the inadequate supply of health professionals in rural areas—the military was faced with a daunting set of entirely new issues.

- The fall of the Berlin Wall in late 1989 brought an end to the Cold War. The military mission shifted from preparedness to fight an all-out war against a monolithic enemy (i.e., the Soviet Union) to engagement of small forces in limited skirmishes on remote and unfamiliar terrain (e.g., Kuwait, Iraq, Bosnia, Macedonia, Dominican Republic).
- The federal government became simultaneously committed to balancing the budget. This sudden change in political climate meant not only the end of supplemental appropriations to

---

TELEMEDICINE IS . . . BEHAVIORAL TELETHERAPY FOR SOLDIERS

If necessity begets invention, then the U.S. Department of Defense is compelled to reinvent military medicine. Our armed forces have been given dramatically different missions and smaller budgets since the end of the Cold War. The resulting challenges and their solutions help define telemedicine for the future, as shown by progressive examples from the Hawaii-based Project AKAMAI (http://www.prpo.tamc.amedd.army.mil).

The shift toward a career force means more married soldiers, but base closures and personnel reductions mean longer deployments away from home. Counseling is often necessary due to the resulting stress on marital and parental relationships and its adverse impact on a soldier's performance, but—catch 22—budget cuts and smaller missions restrict the use of counselors in today's military theaters. Instead, interactive video is being used to connect soldiers in remote areas with mental health professionals at large bases. Members of the soldier's or sailor's family can come to the therapist's office to create a complete, real-time family therapy session. Early results suggest that these video interventions are just as effective as face-to-face counseling.

Sailors are prone to special problems (e.g., claustrophobia, acrophobia, motion sickness) that can be helped by interaction with a qualified psychologist or

cover the accepted practice of over-budget spending, but a smaller military force as well.

- The rapid development of "high-tech" warfare dramatically increased the value of investments in military personnel. For example, training a helicopter pilot now costs half-a-million dollars, which puts special emphasis on protecting human capital as well as human lives.

- An increase in the number, severity, and awareness of natural disasters created the need for many troops to participate in humanitarian assistance. Activities other than war have become a major focus of military planning and deployment.

The old military health system simply did not mesh with new realities. Soldiers were facing more risks in a growing number of remote locations, yet budget cuts meant fewer military hospitals and health professionals to provide care. Military medicine had to be completely redesigned; every assumption had to be reexamined. The old constraints of time and place had become irrelevant, and overcoming them had become critical. (See "Telemedicine is . . . behavioral teletherapy for soldiers" in the box below.)

The military is not constrained by the crazy patchwork quilt of state medical practice acts and reimbursement policy, so the Department of Defense (DOD) is an ideal "test bed" for reinventing healthcare.

---

psychiatrist. Again, interactive video can bring together a land-based therapist and a sailor at sea to deal with the mental problems of life on a ship.

Better understanding of relationships between health status and military preparedness have underscored the need for soldiers to stop smoking or lose weight. Hypnotherapy has demonstrated its effectiveness for smoking cessation and weight loss, but hypnotherapists are simply not going to be found in many new billets. Telehypnosis using video and audio connections is, therefore, being tested as an important tool in the new military health system. Other telemedical interventions are being developed to help deployed troops make positive lifestyle changes for dealing with health problems like obesity, heart disease, and diabetes.

Neuropsychological assessments are occasionally needed to evaluate preparedness of remotely located troops in situations where the presence of mental health professionals would compromise the military mission. Mental health professionals are finding ways to use networked computers and satellite telecommunications to conduct needed assessments.

These models of behavioral teletherapy are still under development, and some problems have been encountered. Nevertheless, networked computers and video cameras are opening a promising new realm of possibilities in a military with a whole new mission.

Recognizing the challenges and opportunities associated with the new environment, military leaders made two other momentous decisions. They decided that the health branches of all four armed services (Army, Air Force, Navy, and Marines) would work together in a unified command, and they decided to work closely and openly with the civilian sector. The headquarters for this command is the Telemedicine and Advanced Technology Research Center (TATRC) at Ft. Detrick, Maryland.[2]

Our organizational analysis may seem a bit detached from the technological focus of this chapter, but we believe the military's refreshingly apolitical approach to telemedicine helps explain its creative leadership. The Department of Defense has been directly or indirectly involved in the development of almost all the technologies to which we now turn our attention, and it deserves special recognition for a job well done. Here are examples of such developments that are starting to define the realm of possibilities for telemedicine.

PERSONAL INFORMATION CARRIERS

The personal information carrier (PIC) is perhaps an ideal item to begin an introduction to the technologies of telemedicine. It embodies all the promise of the telemedicine revolution, from instantly accessible patient information to consumer empowerment. It is being developed by TATRC and private contractors with DOD funds, with great potential for commercial (i.e., civilian) distribution as it moves beyond the research and development stage in the near future. We believe the PIC provides a desirable alternative to interactive video as an emblem of the future of the telemedicine revolution.

The PIC is a multimedia storage device that will contain a patient's entire medical record in a small, easy-to-carry format. It is, in effect, a very dense storage medium packed into a small, convenient package—like a CD-ROM in concept, but much smaller. Prototypes in the development stage are the size and shape of a credit card, a key, a ring, and a military dog tag. (In an early stage of development, PIC was called Medi-Tag because of its resemblance to a dog tag.) Individuals will keep their PICs on key rings, in their wallets, or on a necklace. One or more of the prototypes will ultimately be able to record, store, and transmit an extensive collection of medical data, including text from medical records, diagnostic images, EKG and EEG readings, drug histories, laboratory results, medical warnings, and other clinically relevant information.

The PIC can be inserted into a reader that establishes the electronic link with a computer and the network beyond. The information on a PIC is accessed by "swiping" the device through a credit card reader or inserting it in a special card that fits into a PCMCIA (personal computer memory card/international association) slot, now a standard accessory on almost all computers. Old information can be downloaded and new data entered in seconds. Security can be protected by personal identification numbers (PINs), such as the code we enter when we use our credit cards to withdraw cash at automatic teller machines (ATMs), or by newer devices that read fingerprints or scan retinas.

Anyone who doubts the viability of PIC technology needs to be reminded that cash machines and other ATMs were met with widespread skepticism when introduced in the 1980s. And just as credit card companies keep current accounts of our charges and payments, we will contract with a national medical records company that will maintain all our medical records in a secure, central file. We will also be able to get a new PIC when we need a replacement, and we will be able to direct all our new medical data to the central file so that our record is always up-to-date.

With capacity up to one hundred megabytes of information and no limits on storage capacity in sight, the PIC is obviously a whole lot more than the "smart card" that would have contained the details of our health plan if President Clinton had succeeded with his reforms in 1993–94. It creates a whole new way to think about healthcare because it puts the patient in control of his or her own health information. Further, PIC technology will open healthcare to the new realm of electronic commerce, allowing us to "shop" when the "store" is closed (e.g., to engage in our part of medical transactions at a time and place convenient to us) and to fill our own market baskets before we go through the "check-out" (e.g., to control our consumption based on our health plan and available out-of-pocket resources). By now, you've no doubt got the picture, so use your own imagination to see how healthcare will be different when liberated from the constraints of time and place in a world of instant information.

PERSONAL STATUS MONITORS

One of medical care's major advances in the second half of the twentieth century was development of modern emergency medical services (EMS) systems. Thanks to the creation of paramedics (another military contribution to civilian healthcare) and modern ambulances in the 1960s and 1970s, the lifesaving paradigm shifted from transporting critical patients to the nearest hospital in a refitted hearse to saving lives by bringing life-support care to the scene of the illness or injury. The improvement in outcomes was dramatic, but precious time was still lost while the ambulance was en route.

Researchers in both military and civilian research centers recently began to rethink the problem: why not develop devices that could forewarn of an impending health crisis? For example, medical assistance could be dispatched upon early warning signs, such as a heart monitor that simultaneously issued a warning and dispatched help when the first signs of an abnormal heartbeat were recorded. As an alternative response, corrective devices like pacemakers could be worn to start therapy even before the arrival of qualified health personnel.

This creative line of reasoning has generated research and development projects that will make telemedicine even more powerful. Implantable, wearable, and portable monitoring devices are being designed to provide real-time information about inauspicious changes in vital signs, and some are even linked to devices that provide corrective intervention. Some of the most advanced developments currently find their best uses in the field of home health. Tabletop sensors can monitor blood pressure, cardiac rhythms, blood sugar, and a growing number of other signs that can provide an immediate objective assessment of health status.

TELEMEDICINE IS . . . REMOTE ANALYSIS OF ICU DATA

Imagine the complexity of interactions between state-of-the-art equipment and highly trained health professionals in an intensive care unit (ICU). Nurses monitor the screens of different high-tech devices that track health status of the unit's gravely ill patients. Upon noticing deviations from target parameters, nurses call a doctor to the ICU to interpret the data and decide what should be done to try to reverse the situation.

Although advances in monitoring technology have continually improved the quantity and quality of critical care data over the past twenty years, one thing hasn't changed. Doctors have still been required to come to the hospital to view the monitors—until researchers at UCLA's Neurosurgery ICU realized that networked computers could eliminate the inefficiency of summoning a doctor to the ICU.

Now, thanks to capabilities of TeleTrend software (owned and distributed by Nicolet Biomedical, Inc. (800)356-0007; www.nicoletbiomedical.com) and the World Wide Web (www.bmml.medsch.ucla.edu/teletrend), medical specialists can consult a patient's latest physiological and neurological signs from their homes, offices, or any other location where a computer can be attached to a telephone. The system not only transmits the patient's data; it also allows the screen on the doctor's

These devices only become part of telemedicine when they are linked to a network of health practitioners who can use the information to take care of patients at different times and in different places. However, almost all such devices already are (or will soon be) IP-enabled, meaning they use network communications protocols to ensure that they are "plug and play" compatible with telecomputing systems. Expect to see explosive growth in direct consumer sales of personal status monitors, along with competition among a growing number of telemedicine service providers who will want to be the caregiver at the other end of the line—instantly available, twenty-four hours a day.

ROBOTICS AND NANOTECHNOLOGY

Robotics is the manipulation of task-specific machines (robots) at a distance. When artificial intelligence is embedded in the control system, robots can also operate beyond the typical constraints of time. With telecomputing added to the mix, robotics obviously has potential in the realm of telemedicine. Telemedical robotics is still in its infancy, but the field seems to offer enough promise that it deserves brief mention in our future-oriented analysis.

Early ideas include the development of life-support machines that can be used to find and treat injured persons in dangerous environments.

laptop to emulate the ICU monitors. For example, a neurosurgeon can remotely correlate the patient's heart rate, oxygen saturation, intracranial pressure, and other clinically relevant signs with the monitored neurological data as if he or she were in the ICU with the nurse and the patient.

TeleTrend integrates and synchronizes vital data, allowing doctors to customize display screens and interpret information more rapidly. The system also incorporates specialized analytical tools that improve insight into a patient's overall condition. This application of telemedicine allows one doctor to be virtually in two places at once, and it allows several doctors in different locations to examine the same data and confer with each other in real-time using chat rooms and white-board technology.

The improvements in terms of quality and cost of care are obvious now that a neurospecialist can cover the hospital ICU without leaving the office. Hospitalized patients get attention as if the doctor were present to interpret the data on their ICU monitors, and office patients don't experience long delays while the doctor is unexpectedly called to the hospital. In addition, doctors see more patients at lower overall cost since no time is lost in transit. Even if the only benefit were keeping the doctor on schedule, that would be a revolutionary outcome for all concerned.

An EMS robot might, for example, enter a room where dangerous gasses were accidentally released, locate affected individuals, assess their status, and transport living victims to a safer environment for treatment. Robots might also sort through the rubble left by an explosion or earthquake to find and treat survivors. Home health robots are being designed to support essential activities of daily living, including administration of prescription medications and provision of immediate aid to elderly patients who have fallen.

Nanotechnology, intelligent machines reduced to microscopic size, may have even more to offer in healthcare.[3] Researchers are already exploring the development of very tiny devices that could float in the blood and remove dangerous plaque from coronary arteries, or microchips that could be implanted to monitor biochemical activity and produce corrective drugs *in situ*, such as an "artificial pancreas" to monitor and control the blood sugar of diabetics moment-to-moment.

As already noted, the links between robotics, nanotechnology, and telemedicine may be a bit tenuous as this book is written in 1999, but we are excited by some of the possibilities. We can imagine a day in the future when a patient in Colorado will ingest prescription nano-robots that are programmed by a clinical pharmacist in Illinois who monitors and reprograms the devices over the Internet in response to changes in the patient's condition.

Lest we lose readers who think we have suddenly lapsed into science fiction, we'll return to telemedical technologies that are already moving from R&D into everyday application. But we note in passing that both authors can recollect when people thought that the technology behind pacemakers and injection pumps was too complicated to ever become useful. As for the future of robotics and nanotechnology in telemedicine, just remember you heard it here first.

TELEPRESENCE AND VIRTUAL REALITY

Telepresence is another paradigm-breaking advance that is developing alongside telemedicine. It complements the real-time visual presence established by interactive video (i.e., "talking heads"), adding sensations of physical presence through peripheral devices that are tied to the communications network. For example, a practitioner at one end of a telemedicine consultation can simulate clinical touch by manipulating minute probes on a mechanical input device attached to a distant patient. Resistance, pressure, and other physical characteristics measured by the probes are transmitted back over the network to an output device, such as a mechanical glove worn by the clinician. The clinician feels haptic responses which simulate the sense of touch that would have been experienced if the clinician were actually in physical contact with the patient.

The realistic effects made possible by combining mechanical and information technologies are already familiar to teenagers and a few brave adults who play games at high-tech arcades. Telemedicine will quickly spread clinical applications of the same converging technologies, with some of the most remarkable results coming from the practice of telepresence surgery.

Telepresence surgery allows a surgeon in one location—possibly a medical office, or even a vacation home—to manipulate surgical instruments placed inside a patient located somewhere else. A surgical technician with the patient in the operating area inserts and removes the instruments, ensures sterility, and coordinates physical procedures with the nurse anesthetist or anesthesiologist who is responsible for managing the patient's life functions during the procedure.

How, you might ask, can a surgeon possibly perform an operation without being there to see the patient? Telepresence surgery is not as far-fetched as it may seem because surgeons have been removing gallbladders and repairing knees for years now with scopes inserted into tiny holes and snaked through the body to the surgical site (a process known as minimal access surgery). Surgeons watch the results of their hand movements "amplified" on big screen, high-resolution television monitors. They don't see real tissue during the procedure. Sometimes sitting at consoles across the operating room with their backs to the patient, the surgeons operate on an electronic image. They might as well be miles away, and that is the point of telemedicine.

Telepresence surgery will allow patients with a growing number of medical problems to have their operations performed by nationally recognized specialists, but without traveling across the country to see the doctors in person. Instead, patients will be able to go to local clinics with electronic links to surgeons at national centers of excellence. The technology will allow electronic "shopping," too, as patients give several surgeons the opportunity to review their Web-based medical records (including lab reports and diagnostic images) and make competing proposals to perform the operation.

These new options are made possible in large part by the rapid development of virtual reality (VR).[4] For example, computers can convert the digital record of a computerized tomography (CT) scan of a brain tumor into a three-dimensional (3-D) image.[5] Surgeons can then study the tumor on a video monitor, plan the approach that does the least damage to surrounding tissue, and practice the procedure in a

PIONEERS IN TELEMEDICINE:
JAY H. SANDERS, M.D., F.A.C.P.

Jay Sanders was a resident in internal medicine at Massachusetts General Hospital (MGH) in 1967 when one of his mentors, Dr. Ken Bird, talked about installing an interactive video link between MGH and Logan Airport. It would allow doctors at MGH to see patients at the airport without losing an hour or more in traffic jams that plagued the underwater tunnel between Logan and the city. "I thought it was the dumbest thing I had ever heard," he remembers, "but here I am—32 years later—devoting all my professional effort to that crazy idea."

The Hospital Medical Director, Dr. John Knowles (later to become President of the Rockefeller Foundation), helped give birth to telemedicine by funding the link to Logan. Dr. Sanders completed his residency, left Boston, and joined the faculty at the University of Miami School of Medicine. As director of the medical teaching program and head of the medical intensive care unit (ICU) and the Division of General Medicine at Jackson Memorial Hospital, he did not expect to hear any more about Ken Bird's "crazy idea."

Much to his surprise, Dr. Sanders became personally involved in telemedicine soon after arriving in Florida. He got a grant from the National Science Foundation to study physician maldistribution, and one of the study sites was the Dade County (Florida) Correctional Health System. Telemedicine could solve some of the complicated problems of caring for inmates, so Dr. Sanders established the nation's first telemedicine program for a corrections facility in 1973, working in cooperation with the Westinghouse Electric Corporation.

True to the spirit of the "see one, do one, teach one" medical training model, Dr. Sanders began to promote and use telemedicine whenever possible in his role as a teacher. "I was convinced that telemedicine would become a major part of healthcare because it made sense," he recalls. "It just didn't happen as fast as I expected, but it sure is happening fast now."

He tirelessly promoted telemedicine throughout the 1980s, so he was the logical person to direct a major telemedicine initiative launched by the State of Georgia in 1990. He was concurrently appointed to an endowed chair as Eminent Scholar in Telemedicine at the Medical College of Georgia, and he worked with many groups to establish the state's highly respected system. "The Georgia project was a truly phenomenal experience because so many different organizations worked together to create a system that worked," he proudly notes. (For a summary of this project, see Sanders, JH and FJ Tedesco. "Telemedicine: Bringing Medical Care to Isolated Communities," *Journal of the Medical Association of Georgia* (May, 1993): 237-241.)

Jay got used to a lot of air travel because his wife—a clinical psychologist with a TV show in Miami—and children continued to live in Florida when he went to work in Georgia. He fondly remembers being an occasional guest on his wife's program and talking about his two clinical passions, telemedicine and coronary artery risk factors.

In 1996, Dr. Sanders became President of the American Telemedicine Association and moved to Washington, D.C., to provide political leadership on key issues like reimbursement and program funding. "I think my family thought I was certifiably crazy," he says, because the position was unpaid, so he also established a consulting firm, The Global Telemedicine Group (TGTG), in McLean, Virginia.

The gamble to move to the Washington area paid off because telemedicine is now becoming well-established in federal programs, and TGTG is gaining recognition as a telemedicine services provider. In addition to working as a consultant in all aspects of telemedicine domestically, Dr. Sanders is working with several less-developed countries that see telemedicine as a way to move directly to modern delivery systems.

He is a founding board member and now past president of the American Telemedicine Association. He directs the U.S. telemedicine initiatives with the G-8 nations and serves as Chairman of the Rural Healthcare Committee and member of the Executive Committee of the Universal Service Administration Committee. He has also tirelessly represented the interests of telemedicine with working groups of the Federal Communications Commission, the Institute of Medicine of the National Academy of Sciences, the Department of Defense, the World Health Organization, and the National Library of Medicine.

As the record clearly shows, no one has done more to promote telemedicine at home and abroad. He clearly misses the days when he was a practicing physician and teacher, so he is particularly proud of telemedicine's growing contributions to patient care. "Telemedicine has given us the opportunity to see patients where they are sick, not where the doctor works. Improving our ability to get service to the point of need is a big step forward for medical care. That's why I became a doctor in the first place."

virtual environment before performing the operation—just as a pilot learns to "fly" unfamiliar equipment in a simulator before taking an actual plane on a real flight. Alternatively, a clinical pharmacist could study ways to administer chemotherapeutic agents to the tumor without surgery. Talk about a revolution!

THE INTERNET AND WORLD WIDE WEB

Telemedicine is made possible by the convergence of many technologies, but the Internet (the Net) and the World Wide Web (WWW, or the Web) may be the most powerful among them. The Net and the Web are the catalysts that allow telemedicine's other enabling technologies to move beyond their own spheres and contribute to global change in the world of healthcare. Minimal access surgery (see previous section) illustrates this point. It is a significant advance in surgery in its own right, but minimal access surgery does not break barriers of time and place nor empower consumers until it is integrated into the distributed world of telecomputing.

The growth of the Net and the Web has been explosive. Both have moved from the periphery of telemedicine to center stage in just a few years. Their intertwined future cannot be predicted with certainty. Indeed, the Internet was almost an afterthought when the first outline for this book was submitted to the publisher in late 1996.[6] It merited one line in a subsection about computer networks; the Web wasn't included at all. Together, they are arguably the predominant topic in the book that is finally published less than three years later.

This vignette suggests the possibility of even more surprises in the coming few years. (After all, revolutions are not always controllable.) Several current events need to be taken into consideration by healthcare leaders with responsibility for keeping up with this technology:

- The Internet backbone is being redesigned by a consortium of public and private organizations, and the second generation Net will be widely available early in the twenty-first century. It will be faster and more secure, and it will have much greater capabilities to handle multimedia traffic (e.g., telephony, video, massive databases).
- The "last mile" problem of linking low-bandwith channels (e.g., copper wire) to the Web's high-speed backbone (e.g., fiberoptic cable) will gradually be solved as consumers get direct access to broadband services from their homes and offices via cable and wireless networks.

- The "look and feel" of the Web will be enhanced and its functionality improved by a new approach to programming. Hypertext Markup Language (HTML), the software that is currently used for most Web pages, effectively limits the Web to static images. The new language, Extensible Markup Language (XML), in addition to supporting a much richer slice of virtual reality, will solve many problems associated with hardware and software incompatibility.[7]
- Better computer operating systems and more powerful search engines are expected to be widely distributed beginning in 1999. Users will be able to go directly to desired information faster than ever before. The new systems will eliminate many of the inefficiencies that have hindered use of the Web until now.[8]

Further, the evolution of telemedicine on the Internet will almost certainly be affected—probably for the better—and accelerated by start-up companies and by mergers of existing leaders in the industry.[9] The Internet was started with funds from the federal government (predominantly the Defense Advanced Research Projects Agency, or DARPA), but private investments are beginning to generate incredible growth in companies that provide Web-based telemedical services.

The changes are coming so fast that we see no value in providing more extensive information about telemedicine on the Internet in a book finished in the summer of 1999. Details about specific companies, operating systems, interfaces, and applications would be out-of-date long before the book is out-of-print. Our approach is to provide readers with information that is likely to have a longer half-life, that is, a list of practical recommendations for planning telemedicine services and making appropriate investments in technology. However, before concluding this chapter with our list of specific recommendations, we explore the basic technological issues in the context of interactive video.

INTERACTIVE VIDEO

As shown at the beginning of this book, telemedicine was basically synonymous with interactive video until just a few years ago. We've identified other technologies that have expanded and enriched telemedicine since then, but interactive video has not disappeared. Nor will it disappear in the future. It will continue to be used in clinical situations where real-time, face-to-face interaction is necessary. In addition, interactive video will likely remain an important technology for some nonclinical uses such as administrative meetings and continuing professional education.

Its use may even increase somewhat in other areas as costs are lowered by advances in supportive technologies. Interactive video is the most expensive modality overall because it involves many resources, so our overview of interactive video is a good place to begin exploring technical and economic aspects of most forms of telemedicine.

Bandwidth and Signal Quality

Bandwidth is a conceptual measure of the amount of information that can be transmitted through a communications channel in a second. It quantifies the amount of information that can be "pushed" through a "pipe." The bigger the pipe, the bigger the bandwidth. It is measured most commonly in bits per second (bps), kilobits per second (Kbps), or megabits per second (Mbps). Fiberoptic cable, for example, can carry more bps that regular telephone line, so fiber is said to have more (broader) bandwidth than copper.

Video demands more bandwidth than other technologies of telemedicine because so much information needs to be transmitted to form a moving image on a monitor. Details regarding the picture and its size, colors, and movement from frame to frame all need to be sent over the cable or broadcast band that connects the receiver (monitor)

TELEMEDICINE IS . . . KIDNEY DIALYSIS WITH INTERACTIVE VIDEO

Thanks to the dedicated efforts of nephrologist Jack Moncrief, M.D., local care for end-stage renal disease (ESRD) has been available for many years to kidney failure patients in rural Giddings, Texas. However, the nature of the doctor-patient relationship was changed dramatically in the early 1990s when the Texas Telemedicine Project installed an interactive video link over the fifty-five miles between the dialysis center in Giddings and Dr. Moncrief's office in Austin.

Before telemedicine, Dr. Moncrief spent at least three hours per week of "windshield time" just to get to the rural dialysis center. Each of the twenty-five to thirty patients in Giddings got an average of five minutes of the doctor's time. Several had to drive back up to Austin when they had special problems. Only the few lucky patients being dialyzed on the day of the doctor's visit got to see him during treatment. And Dr. Moncrief had to spend many hours waiting at the nursing station between appointments.

Now, with telemedicine, Dr. Moncrief stays in Austin and schedules a live, face-to-face meeting with each patient during his or her dialysis session in

and transmitter (camera, VCR, etc.). Making the video image bigger, sharper, or smoother require more bandwidth. Faster is not an issue. Electrons and photons travel at the same speed, regardless of the quality of the underlying image.

Bandwidth is not free. Fiberoptic cable has the capacity to create top-quality video at 30 frames per second (fps) on a 35" monitor, but at a high cost. Ubiquitous standard telephone lines—called "twisted pairs" or "copper pairs" in technical jargon—can carry a video signal at a much lower cost. However, the picture transmitted over the phone will be small (3.5" screen) and jerky (15 fps) because telephone lines cannot carry enough information to recreate a big, sharp, and smooth video image.

Given this trade-off between quality and cost, the key economic issue is to match bandwidth to the application. A telephone-based video system is acceptable for many home health needs, for example. Watching a patient take a pill or looking for health hazards in his or her kitchen can be done just fine on a small screen with slightly jerky motion. On the other hand, lots of bandwidth is required for telepresence surgery.

Unfortunately, telemedicine in its early years developed a reputation for being expensive because early adopters used dedicated, broadband video networks for jobs that did not require moving images or high resolution. Almost all early telemedicine projects incurred the expense of maintaining a lot of bandwidth for video, but a very high

Giddings. When patients want a confidential consultation with the doctor, they can go to a private room equipped for two-way exchanges. The patients' local doctors in Giddings and other specialists in Austin can also join the virtual visit when indicated.

The published studies of this innovative telemedicine project suggest the changes were for the better for all concerned. (Moncrief, JW. "Telemedicine in the Care of the End-Stage Renal Disease Patient," *Advances in Renal Replacement Therapy* 5(4):286, 291 (October 1998). By eliminating waits between appointments and automobile travel, the doctor's time to see the same number of patients dropped by approximately fourteen hours per week, and many patient trips to Austin were eliminated because interactive video consultations could be arranged on days when Dr. Moncrief was not scheduled to come to Giddings. Perhaps most importantly, patient response is enthusiastic and appreciative. They can all see the doctor during their dialysis appointment; no one has to return to the center on a different day when "the doctor is in."

percentage of clinical needs—the vast majority, in the authors' opinion—can be met with inexpensive, narrowband approaches like store-and-forward transmission of fixed images over the Internet.

Telemedicine will prosper as decision makers learn to match the bandwidth with the task. Applications that used to be done on interactive video will migrate to less-expensive platforms, thus ending much of telemedicine's high-cost reputation. Eventually (within a decade, we believe), the enormous investment in competing high-bandwidth technologies will afford almost universal access to fast information pipes, and bandwidth will cease to be a critical factor in systems planning.

Platforms and Compression

As originally planned, this book was going to include a table comparing the bandwidth of different pipes. However, such technical detail is becoming less relevant. Telemedical interactions that required a really big pipe only a year ago can now be accomplished with smaller bandwidth. Engineers and programmers have effectively learned how to push more information through a pipe of a given size. We believe that such progress will continue and have decided against including a table that would be quickly outdated. The important point is that bandwidth is declining as a bottleneck in the growth of telemedicine.

Several factors contribute to the capability to push more information through a pipe of fixed bandwidth.

- Compression allows many images to be recreated at the receiving end with smaller data sets. Without compression, every little detail of an image must be transmitted for each consecutive frame. With compression, image elements that do not change from frame to frame (such as a fixed background) are not transmitted. Compression within each frame, such as representing uniform areas with abbreviated code, further reduces the data load.

- Better switches allow bits of data to flow in and out of the pipe at faster rates, and faster routers redirect the data to intended destinations with increasing speed. Connections between pipes can now be made at speeds that were unimaginable only a few years ago, and progress in switching is expected to continue.

- As more data are acquired digitally, transmission systems do not have to take the time to translate analog information into digital form before sending it through the pipe (and then reconverting the digital signal back to analog at the receiving end). Also, eliminating analog-to-digital conversion allows systems to use less electrical power, and all-digital systems are many times faster than the predominantly analog systems initially used in telemedicine.

In addition, engineers have gotten much better at connecting different types of pipe. In the early days of telemedicine—that is, until about 1998—systems tended to be built primarily with the same type of pipe. The ideal network consisted of fiberoptic cable from one end to the other, and some proposed telemedicine projects were never implemented for lack of a complete fiberoptic link.

Technologies have recently been developed to link several different data pipes, and interconnectedness is becoming common. For example, a diagnostic image might start its digital trip on a copper telephone line, be shunted onto a satellite system for transmission across the country, be downloaded to a local area network via microwave, and finally be delivered to a radiologist's office over a fiberoptic ring within the hospital. Significant cost savings are achieved because newer technologies can create a coherent data path with existing, but different, platforms. Sadly, the potential of telemedicine is underestimated by people who do not know that technological advances have reduced or eliminated problems of connectivity.

Technical Standards and Networks

Happily, the future of interconnectedness is being enhanced by the development of common technical standards for hardware, software, and data. The bits of information flowing out of different pipes were frequently incompatible in the past, but they are increasingly being converted to the technical equivalents of least-common denominators. Shared standards enhance the flow of information along a varied path, and telemedicine benefits accordingly.

The development of Internet Protocol (IP), an evolving set of shared standards that allow different systems to communicate over the Internet, has been a particularly significant boon to the development of integrated networks. IP-enabled applications all "speak the same language," regardless of the machine on which they originated or the mode of transmission. Within the medical field, standard nomenclatures such as SNOMED and HL-7 are further reducing the burdens of achieving interconnectivity.

The movement toward shared technical standards helps give incredible vitality to telemedicine. Thanks to the technical and political skills of electrical engineers and computer system designers, telemedicine is quickly overcoming problems associated with it when telemedicine was synonymous with interactive video. Shared standards and networks have proven their value as solutions, and the resulting gains in interconnectivity will accelerate the pace of the telemedicine revolution. Long live open systems!

Y2K

Before examining the keys to success, we must briefly mention a major roadblock on the road to telemedicine—the millennium bug, or Y2K. Very substantial resources in the healthcare industry are focused on ensuring that medical equipment and software will not malfunction at midnight on December 31, 1999, because internal system clocks assume that the next day is January 1, 1900.

Addressing the Y2K problem has diverted a lot of money that might otherwise have been spent on telemedicine projects. The good news is that the problem will not last for long after the turn-of-the-millennium. A few disasters will likely occur for health systems or medical equipment manufacturers that did not take proper preventive measures, but the vast majority of healthcare providers will start the year 2000 with minimal problems. Y2K should quickly disappear as a drain on budgets, thus liberating money for investments in telemedicine.

TELEMEDICINE IS . . . A MEDICAL SCHOOL DERMATOLOGY CLASS

Medical education certainly illustrates the long-standing constraints of space and time in healthcare. Without so much as a second thought, we expect medical students and professors to come together in a classroom or operating theater in order to view slides, hear a lecture, study a cadaver, or examine a patient. The schedule dictates that class must go on at a predetermined time and place—even if equally important activities like patient care, lab work, or sleep are interrupted.

Professors in the Department of Dermatology at the Indiana University Medical School in Indianapolis are pioneering the use of telemedicine to improve the situation for all concerned. Using a software platform licensed by WebCT (http://webct.com), the faculty has put the introductory dermatology course on the Web. Now, students can see textbook-quality photographs of different skin problems on their own computer screens and study accompanying text whenever convenient to them. They can test their knowledge by reviewing quiz questions built into the virtual course and take exams on their own computers whenever they are ready.

Customized links give medical students direct access to on-line archives and dermatology case files of the pathology department. For example, a student who

With Y2K out of the way, telemedicine's growth should accelerate dramatically in 2000 and beyond.

KEYS TO SUCCESS IN TELEMEDICINE

Rapid technological progress explains why telemedicine's realm of possibilities is expanding at such an amazing rate. We would, therefore, be doing a disservice to our readers if we were to present static rules for developing telemedicine programs. Instead, we propose several general guidelines for dealing with the evolving technologies of telemedicine.

> ***Stay informed and open-minded.*** This recommendation probably goes without saying because telemedicine is the product of such rapid technological change. Problems that plagued previous telemedical systems are often resolved in a matter of months, and new applications can come to market just as fast. Something that was "true" of telemedicine last year is quite likely to be different now and altogether irrelevant next year. Therefore, preconceived notions should be avoided.
>
> We emphasize the constant need to update and reexamine knowledge about telemedicine because we have talked with many people who rejected telemedicine for the right reasons in the past . . . and then continued to ignore it on the assumption

wants to learn more about a particular skin problem can go to in-depth cases like "a 23-year-old man with itchy wrists" or "a 47-year-old woman with a nodular mass on her flank." The case files include numerous photographs, diagrams, tissue slides, and descriptive commentary to provide in-depth, multidisciplinary information for informed diagnosis and treatment.

Telemedical dermatology education allows the professors to update their teaching materials at any time, thus solving the problem of traditional textbooks and handouts that are costly to revise and quickly dated (even though recently printed). The professors have also begun to link their dermatology course to the school's Continuing Medical Education Division so that practicing doctors can get credit for updating their skills in dermatology.

The on-line courses are being translated into Spanish and Portuguese, which demonstrates yet another way in which telemedicine is crossing frontiers. Thanks to this pioneering work being done by dermatology professors at the University of Indiana School of Medicine, telemedicine is transcending not only space and time, but culture and language as well.

that little or nothing has changed. We like to tell people that telemedicine is changing so fast that it takes us—experts in the field—an incredible amount of time and effort just to stay confused. If we have accomplished one goal with this book, we hope that we have made a compelling argument to keep giving telemedicine another look. Forget any notions of a "steady state" technology.

Practitioners, executives, planners, and other healthcare decision makers must constantly renew their knowledge about telemedicine if they expect their enterprises to thrive in the twenty-first century. The Websites identified in Chapter 8 are a great place to pursue this quest because they will be updated frequently to reflect the rapid evolution of telemedicine. Attending major programs and trade shows, such as the annual meetings of the American Telemedicine Association and the Association of Telemedicine Service Providers (see Chapter 8 for details) will be additionally helpful, probably even essential, for professionals with organizational responsibility for telemedicine.

We have one very important corollary for readers who are not yet computer-literate: *learn to use the Internet and the World Wide Web ASAP!* Fluency in telecomputing will be an essential basic skill for anyone who hopes to thrive in the world of twenty-first century healthcare. Being wired and on-line won't be an option much longer; it is rapidly becoming a precondition for surviving the telemedicine revolution. For senior executives, delegating electronic communications to subordinates will be increasingly self-destructive. If you need a little extra motivation to join the telecomputing revolution, you can safely assume that all your competitors and most of your customers will be Internet-enabled by 2001, if not sooner. Enough said.

Specify the need, then select the technology. Technology can do some really cool things, but it can also waste a lot of resources and acquire a bad reputation if it becomes a part of the problem rather than a solution. As we've previously noted, technology is nothing more than a tool to facilitate a specific process; it should never dictate the process. Telemedicine's reputation still suffers in some quarters because early adopters often installed hardware, usually an interactive video system funded by a big grant, and then tried to figure out what to do with it.

Expensive and unpleasant learning experiences can be avoided in the future if telemedicine is adopted to meet a carefully defined need. Decision makers should start by identifying a specific job that needs to be done or done better, such as improving access to specialists, eliminating drug medication errors, providing more complete medical records to clinicians, treating patients in their homes, collecting information about consumer behavior, etc. Then, the technologies of telemedicine should be evaluated, along with other possible approaches, to identify the optimal response.

Telemedicine will not always be the right answer, but we believe it will quickly become the solution of choice for a large number of problems. However, the problem to be addressed must be clearly defined first, and telemedicine should be evaluated with respect to a full range of options that will often include human resources (e.g., retraining displaced workers, hiring new workers to meet growing demand) as well as technology.

Base investments on money saved, not money spent. Once clinicians and administrators identify telemedicine as the best way to meet a specific need, financial managers will inevitably enter the picture. Their traditional approach to financial analysis is not always relevant to the realities of today's new technologies, so some real problems can arise at this critical juncture. Many pieces of telemedicine equipment will be technologically obsolete long before they are fully amortized. The accountants may, therefore, oppose a clinically and competitively desirable investment just because it does not "pencil out at the bottom line."

This book is not the place for discussing new approaches to cost accounting for a high-tech era.[10] However, leaving aside the possible justification for defensive investments—expenditures that must be made because competitors have made them—our experience leads us to conclude that healthcare financial analysts must adapt traditional models to the realities of a technological revolution or get out of the way. Old accounting approaches based on direct returns can be counterproductive.

Investments in telemedicine will often need to be justified indirectly by the money they save in other areas. For example, an electronic medical records system would commonly cost more than the labor it replaces, but returns on the investment could include improvements in diagnostic decisions, reductions in

PIONEERS IN TELEMEDICINE:
JEAN-PIERRE THIERRY, M.D.

Try to identify European leaders in telemedicine, and the name of Dr. Jean-Pierre Thierry invariably comes to the fore. Whether through literature searches or personal inquiries, his name is mentioned far more than any other. He has gained this prominence over the past decade by managing a wide variety of public and private ventures throughout Europe under the banner of Symbion, the consulting firm he manages from his office in Maisons Lafitte, a small town on the outskirts of Paris.

A physician known for his special interests in the socioeconomic and political dimensions of healthcare delivery, Dr. Thierry was commissioned in 1991 by three departments of the French government (Health, Industry, and Research) to prepare a detailed analysis of *télémédecine,* a subject that was just beginning to enter discussions at the cabinet level. His report emphasized the need to use technology to improve the quality of communications between health professionals, and it explored other nontechnical dimensions of telemedicine.

The 1993 government report became the basis of a 90-minute prime-time special on French television, which generated many invitations to give lectures on telemedicine to groups of health professionals in France and several other countries. A consortium of 15 companies also hired Dr. Thierry to create a "virtual hospital" and technology showroom in Paris. It was visited by health professionals from throughout Europe during its two years of existence.

The basic concept of the virtual hospital has influenced an ongoing project funded by the European Union and directed by Dr. Thierry. He has also designed and managed several telemedicine projects in France, including current work to create a perinatal network that will directly involve pregnant women in the management of their own pregnancies through regional intranets. Similar projects are underway in other European countries, so Dr. Thierry does a lot of foreign travel.

His extensive writings focus on the overall benefits that should be expected from the convergence of telecommunications and informatics. He shuns the idea of technology for technology's sake, and he puts particular emphasis on the need to formalize the purpose and organization of healthcare programs before making major investments in technology.

His philosophical and pragmatic approach to the development of telemedicine is not surprising, given that most European countries put a very high priority on preserving universal coverage and comprehensive health insurance. Any radical new concept like telemedicine is initially met with skepticism in Europe because it might threaten the egalitarian foundation of national health plans. Government ministries exercise strong control over budgets for telemedicine, so the overall evolution of telemedicine is likely to be slower in Europe than in the United States.

Dr. Thierry believes that some of Europe's most advanced applications of telemedicine are found in Finland, Sweden, and Norway. Like the United States, these three Scandinavian nations have large underserved rural areas, and they are also home to some of the world's leading telecommunications companies (e.g., Nokia, Ericcson). He notes that these countries follow industrial policies designed specifically to promote the implementation of high-tech solutions like telemedicine.

Dr. Thierry's European work constantly involves managing the trade-offs between innovators' needs for flexibility to create new systems and politicians' needs to preserve traditional delivery mechanisms. He must often deal with the difficulties of funding new ventures under these circumstances, but as shown by his extensive list of publications and project reports, he has been successful in showing that the new technologies of telemedicine do not need to conflict with the goals of established national health systems. He notes happily that the European Union's latest healthcare initiative for the information society, Information Society for the Citizens, will include several telemedicine projects to bring medical information directly to patients.

Having visited telemedicine projects in the United States, Dr. Thierry sees major differences in privacy concerns on opposite sides of the Atlantic. European countries tend to place strict controls on any information about individuals. Like most Europeans, Dr. Thierry expresses concerns about Americans' more relaxed attitude toward confidentiality, and he believes that some otherwise excellent telemedicine systems from the United States might be rejected abroad solely because they do not meet European standards for protecting privacy.

Dr. Thierry will continue to negotiate diplomatic *rapprochement* between telemedicine in Europe and North America, but we hope he will never lose his uniquely Gallic approach in the process. France rightly prides itself as the world's leader in serious comics—*bandes désinées,* or B.D., in French—so Dr. Thierry has published an entertaining introduction to telemedicine in comic book form. He is also one of France's experts on American cinema, having given John Baxter the idea of writing his biography on the late Stanley Kubrick. With such eclectic interests, Dr. Thierry fits easily into the list of pioneers who are shaping the future of telemedicine from diverse backgrounds and interests.

medication errors, elimination of duplicated tests, enhancements to continuity of care, and collection of consumer-oriented marketing information. In economic terms, technology-responsive accounting must encompass all the externalities, not just the costs.

Admittedly, telemedicine developed a persistent "high-cost, low-return" reputation from interactive video. Early projects were heavily subsidized by grants, and quite a few were terminated or reduced in scope when the grants expired. The good news is that telemedicine is now much more than interactive video and the costs of the new technologies are falling fast, but the bad news is that many reimbursement and investment policies are still based on assumptions derived from the video era. (This problem is explored in depth in the next chapter.) Telemedicine's champions will have to work hard to make sure that investment decisions are made with respect to the future, not the past.

Always consider outsourcing. An important related issue is answering the "make versus buy" question, that is, deciding whether to purchase resources to do the work internally or to contract with an outside vendor. The right answer will increasingly be to "buy" due to recent growth in the number of specialized telemedicine service providers. These companies make the capital investment in high-capacity telecomputing systems and then sell prepackaged services to many different providers, somewhat like the function performed by hospital purchasing cooperatives that buy large quantities in bulk at considerable volume discounts and then distribute smaller lots to members.

Indeed, growth in the telemedicine services provider business should greatly aid the overall development of telemedicine because it allows healthcare organizations to buy only the services they need. They can also lease capital equipment, such as home health monitoring modules or small portions of a broadband communications line, from specialized companies. The problem of excess capacity is greatly diminished, if not altogether eliminated.

One of the service providers' fastest growing product lines is virtual provider networks (VPN). These vendors incur the costs of establishing a complete telecommunications network, from servers to software and security, and assume the responsibility for upgrading the network as new technology emerges. VPNs respond directly to the cost concerns of the financial managers.

> The health care industry is reaching the same conclusion as every other: technological developments are outpacing many companies' ability to get a return on their investment before the technology becomes obsolete. So out-sourcing network functions to a service provider that delivers the same level of performance as dedicated, private networks—hence the term virtual private—leaves technology upgrading issues in the vendor's court.[11]

The same thinking applies to the use of consultants. Many healthcare providers can "buy" decision-making expertise from consultants at a lower price than they can "make" it with their own employees—as long as the consultants are qualified, experienced, and accountable. With the advantages of specialization in mind, some national consulting firms and software developers are forming joint ventures that specialize in adapting established software platforms to the special needs (e.g., building integrated databases, mining the data, entering the world of electronic commerce) of a wide variety of healthcare organizations. Using consultants should be one of the options considered for starting a telemedicine program because it allows market entrants to benefit from the experience of specialists who have developed, installed, and used the underlying systems.

When buying technology, give careful consideration to commercial off-the-shelf (COTS) systems. Developing customized hardware and software from scratch is expensive, time-consuming, and fraught with glitches. Any decision to undertake do-it-yourself development must be supported by a very compelling reason, such as a mission-critical task that no vendor could come close to fulfilling. Using less-than-perfect COTS systems with good support from a reputable and committed vendor will almost always produce better results than efforts to produce a perfect system on your own.

Insist on user-friendly systems. The development of telemedicine has unquestionably been hindered by early systems that were inconvenient or otherwise hard to use. For example, doctors often had to go to a special telemedicine suite at an odd time (especially common when the video network was shared with daytime educational programs like distance-learning) or had to learn complicated technical procedures in order to use the equipment.

Since the research literature on early telemedicine confirms that many projects were seriously hindered by a cumbersome interface between people and technology, success in the future obviously depends on the development of devices and systems that adapt to humans. The more humans have to adapt to the technology, the less the chances for a successful telemedicine application.

We feel rather strongly about this point. Easy-to-use should be a prerequisite in the selection of equipment and systems for telemedicine. The technology should be intuitive, understandable, graphic, and fast—in other words, user-friendly. It must enhance, not hinder, the process of healthcare. If it slows things down enough to be an annoyance to the users, it probably isn't worth the money because it will not be used.

Consequently, patients and health professionals who are going to use the telemedicine equipment should have an opportunity to try it out before a financial commitment is made. Vendors should also be asked to provide the names of existing customers, and these references should be contacted. Site visits to see the equipment in action are also worthwhile. If checking references and visiting established sites is not possible because brand-new technology is being considered, the purchase contract or lease should place the vendor substantially at-risk for on-time installation and specified performance. Joint ventures between developer/vendors and early users (known as beta-sites in tech-speak, or "guinea pigs" in everyday English) are sometimes worth exploring, as long as the new system truly meets the user's needs and the user gets a fair share of the financial rewards of a successful project.

"User-friendly" also has physical dimensions. For example, equipment used by elderly patients should be big and sturdy, with large and easy-to-read displays and adjustable volume controls for sound interfaces. Patients should have the ability to mute the microphone for privacy when desired.[12]

When a visual image is involved, the background of the health professional's location should have a professional appearance. Locating cameras to ensure eye contact is also very important, and using a substitute examiner can help overcome the absence of "touch capability" (e.g., a home health nurse who touches the patient and reports findings to a remote doctor).[13]

In other words, the technology of telemedicine needs to become transparent because the "gee whiz" factor that attracts users to cool new technologies doesn't last long. If users are not comfortable in their respective roles, they will understandably resist the Seventh Revolution. Fortunately, much user-friendly equipment is now available or being developed, so healthcare professionals and organizations need not make sacrifices with this critical success factor.

Build on open architecture. The Internet has quickly become the communications backbone of telemedicine. Since network computing will likely become even more robust in the foreseeable future, purchasers should only buy telemedicine equipment that is Internet-enabled, even when it will only be used on an exclusively internal network (known as an intranet). The underlying technical concept is *open architecture,* meaning that devices made by one manufacturer are capable of communicating with devices made by other manufacturers because all data can be exported in the common format of the Internet.

The alternative is closed architecture, meaning systems that use proprietary communications protocols and are not readily compatible with devices from original equipment manufacturers (OEM). Some excellent systems were built on closed architecture before the Internet became established, but we have difficulty seeing how they will maintain a competitive position in the future. Closed systems can effectively force users to layer new technology on top of old because all equipment must be purchased from one vendor. In contrast, systems built on open architecture are far more flexible, and users are free to buy competitively and to "mix and match" equipment from different vendors.

Involve the customer. Last, and definitely not least, we remind our readers that telemedicine's ultimate promise is to empower consumers by giving them access to information and, by extension, informed choice in an increasingly competitive market for healthcare services. Telemedicine will ultimately break down geographic and product barriers just as surely as it has already started to liberate the patient-practitioner relationship from traditional constraints of time and place.

A sentinel warning is implied in the recent words of George Whitesides, PhD, a chemistry professor at Harvard:

> The Internet brings the capability for people globally to talk to one another about their medical care in ways they haven't done before. I think one of the interesting possibilities is that the conventional medical system might lose control . . . to groups of patients—groups of people who are ill, talking to one another and convincing themselves that the alternatives lie elsewhere than in the clinical system.[14]

We believe the possibility of this scenario is remote, but it certainly could happen if health professionals and delivery systems try to prevent or control consumer empowerment through telemedicine. The vastly preferable alternative is professional leadership in the telemedicine revolution, with full and active consumer participation. Therefore, in conclusion, we suggest that a collaborative approach to telemedicine—one that *actively* solicits consumer involvement—is among the most important keys to success.

To update and paraphrase one of our country's original revolutionary leaders, healthcare practitioners and delivery systems must become their customers' Internet portal or die. They must determine what their customers want to know, and then they must give them this information. If they fail to act, the vacuum will be filled by well-funded national organizations like drkoop.com or webmd.com. This is a widespread revolution. The competition is no longer local. We must all learn to live with it.

NOTES

1. Detailed descriptions of these programs are provided in the *Federal Telemedicine Directory, 1998* (Department of Health and Human Services, Health Resources and Services Administration, Office for the Advancement of Telehealth). This print document is based on the information contained in an excellent on-line resource, the Federal Telemedicine Gateway, www.tmgateway.org.

2. Interested readers should regularly visit TATRC's Website, www.tatrc.org. It provides an extensive amount of information about the Department of Defense's activities in healthcare in general and telemedicine in particular. Some of the latest technological advances, such as virtual reality applications and trauma simulation for educational purposes, are regularly featured, along with the results of research on both the clinical and economic dimensions of telemedicine. The site is updated regularly and includes useful links to other resources. TATRC was originally named the Military Advanced Technology Management Office (MATMO).

3. For a good general introduction to nanotechnology, see the articles in "Special Report: Nanotechnology" in *Technology Review, MIT's Magazine of Innovation* (March–April, 1999).

4. Readers who are interested in detailed descriptions of the state-of-the-art in VR are referred to Westwood, JD, HM Hoffman, RA Robb, D Stredney (eds.). *Medicine Meets Virtual Reality: The Convergence of Physical and Informational Technologies / Options for a New Era in Healthcare* (Amsterdam &Washington, D.C./Burke, Va.: IOS Press, 1999). This book contains dozens of examples of established and developing applications.

5. An excellent explanation of this application of virtual reality is presented in Grimson, WEL, R Kikinis, FA Jolesz, and PM Black. "Image-Guided Surgery" *Scientific American* (June, 1999): 63–69. The article's footnotes cite several Web sites with supportive graphics:
http://www.ai.mit.edu/projects/medical-vision/;
http://splweb.bwh.harvard.edu:8000; and
http://cisstweb.cs.jhu.edu/

6. We do not think this oversight was unique to the authors. The outline was based on a review of topics covered in existing books and articles on telemedicine, and it was reviewed by several leaders in the field before it was submitted with the original book proposal. No one suggested that more attention be given to the Internet and the WWW, so we think the speed and force of their growth caught just about everyone by surprise.

7. Bosak, J and T Bray. "XML and the Second-Generation Web" *Scientific American* (May 1999): 89–93.

8. Members of the Clever Project. "Hypersearching the Web" *Scientific American* (June 1999): 54–60. This article will be particularly helpful to readers who would like to understand the workings of search engines (e.g., Lycos, Alta Vista, Excite).

9. For example, the merger of Healthaeon and WebMD was announced the week that this section was being written. These two major companies have complementary products, so the merger has considerable potential for synergy if it is managed effectively.

10. The topic of new approaches to investment analysis is regularly covered in the weekly periodicals that specialize in information technology. For example, see the articles in the special section, "Return on Investment," in *Information Week* (May 24, 1999).

11. Guy, S. "Virtual Private Networks" *American Medical News* (March 1, 1999): 26.

12. Private communications with Samuel G. Burgiss, Ph.D., Manager of the Telemedicine and Bioengineering Center, University of Tennessee Medical Center at Knoxville.

13. Moncrief, J. "Telemedicine in the Care of the End-Stage Renal Disease Patient," *Advances in Renal Replacement Therapy* 5(4):288–289 (October 1998).

14. Mitka, M. "Futurists See Longer, Better Life in the Third Millennium," *Journal of the American Medical Association* 281(18):1686 (May 12, 1999).

7

CHAPTER

Issues and Policies of Telemedicine

Telemedicine will not prosper simply because it is a good idea. Like any revolutionary force, telemedicine will encounter considerable resistance as it moves from the fringe to the mainstream of healthcare over the coming years. Deciding whether and how to pay for it, who is qualified to do it, and how to assess its quality are already major issues. Additional concerns will undoubtedly emerge. Payors, practitioners, purchasers, politicians, patients, and representatives of many other special interest groups will become involved in ongoing debates to shape the public policies under which telemedicine will evolve.

This chapter summarizes the current status of the major issues and presents our analysis of key points. With respect to issues related to government, we address the federal perspective because this book is written for a national audience. Readers are reminded that many state governments are involved in setting policies for telemedicine. State laws and regulations will not always be identical to the corresponding federal guidelines. Federal laws can set floors or ceilings for state action—that is, minimum standards that state law must meet but can exceed, or maximum limits that prohibit states from taking more stringent positions. Readers may want to seek additional information about their state's policies to complement the national perspective presented in this book.[1] Of course, issues and policies regarding telemedicine also vary as greatly from country to country as do national health systems themselves.

REIMBURSEMENT FOR TELEMEDICINE

The first question asked in most discussions of telemedicine is, "How will health plans pay for it?" Practitioners and patients alike seem attracted to the promise of telemedicine, but they are concerned that services will not be reimbursed by their health plans. Understandably, fear of unreimbursed expenses is a significant impediment to widespread acceptance of telemedicine, so we will address it first.

For at least two reasons, the long-run impact of the fear of not getting reimbursed is probably overstated. At the very least, it needs to be put in proper perspective.

- First, as shown in Chapter 5's discussions of health insurance and empowered consumers, overall responsibility for payment is being shifted to patients. Out-of-pocket payments are increasing for almost all medical services. Telemedicine is arriving on the scene at a time when health insurance is paying less for just about everything. No one should expect that telemedicine will be fully covered because full coverage for any health service is fast becoming a thing of the past. In addition, we have already suggested that a growing number of consumers will be willing to pay their own money for telemedicine services because they want the choice and the convenience it provides. The telemedicine revolution will be fueled in no small part by money out of peoples' pockets, so health plan resistance is probably overrated as a barrier in the long run.

- Second, the reimbursement problem is a moot point under pure capitation. Health plans that charge a prospectively fixed, per-member, per-month (PMPM) premium do not have to worry about fee-for-service payments when practitioners and provider organizations are also at risk, so telemedicine is very attractive when it can be acceptably substituted for face-to-face care at lower cost. Indeed, some of the most progressive civilian applications of telemedicine have come from Kaiser-Permanente and other capitated, staff-model health plans. The growth of telemedicine will be accelerated by growth in capitation. The problem of paying for telemedicine is concentrated on the fee-for-service side of the medical marketplace, and this side is shrinking.

Nevertheless, government pays close to 45 percent of all health-care bills, and government agencies are not embracing telemedicine as a solution to major problems of our healthcare delivery system. Many private health plans follow the lead set by Medicare, so the future of third-party payment for telemedicine in general is directly affected by Medicare's approach to reimbursement—which is determined by the Health Care Financing Administration (HCFA) under legislative authority from Congress. An inquiry into the current situation suggests that Medicare policy is hindering the evolution of telemedicine.

Medicare does pay for some telemedical services. However, the scope of covered benefits is very limited, the restrictions on payment are stringent, and the pace for developing Medicare policy is extremely slow. Current policy is firmly rooted in HCFA's general rule that healthcare services can only be reimbursed when provided in a face-to-face, in-person encounter between patient and practitioner.[2] This policy was set to prevent reimbursement for telephone consultation decades before telemedicine became a reality, but its defenders are resisting the obvious implications of the Seventh Revolution.

No one should be surprised that a few branches of government are defending the status quo of paying for healthcare. Bureaucracies have a history of fighting change. However, we hasten to add that resistance to change in healthcare is not pervasive in our federal government. As mentioned earlier, some of the most progressive leadership in developing and implementing telemedicine has been provided by government agencies such as the Department of Defense and the National Aeronautics and Space Administration, and several of telemedicine's prominent pioneers are federal employees.

HCFA is the most visible interface between old payment policy and new medical reality. The Healthcare Financing Administration is often given considerable power to set policy because Congress does not want to provide clear direction. That is, Congress passes a well-intentioned law with politically popular objectives, such as cutting the federal deficit. It then delegates to agencies like HCFA the task of making politically unpopular decisions required to implement the law, such as how spending will be cut.

However, in the case of setting policy to reimburse telemedicine, the fundamental problem is probably misdirected legislative intent. The Congressional mandate on reimbursing telemedicine is clearer than usual, and it is already outdated even though it was passed less than two years ago as part of the Balanced Budget Act of 1997. HCFA must follow the general confines of BBA-97, which it does in the following interpretation of the law's authorization to pay for telemedical services only in Rural Health Professional Shortage Areas (HPSA):

> We do not consider a teleconsultation to be a new medical service; rather, we consider it to be a new way or process of delivering a consultation . . . a teleconsultation is equivalent to a traditional, face-to-face consultation only if it permits the consultant to control the examination of the patient as the examination is taking place. With store-and-forward technology, the consultant is reviewing an examination that has already occurred and is limited to whatever information was recorded at that time. We believe that a teleconsultation instead must be an interactive patient encounter.[3]

HCFA's traditional way of thinking is obviously at odds with this book's position that telemedicine constitutes a revolution in medical practice. Unfortunately, a politically polarized Congress could not see beyond balancing the budget when it passed the budget law and disbanded at the end of the 1997 session; it definitely did not authorize the payment agency to entertain new thoughts about medical care. Congress effectively forced HCFA to head in the dubious direction of modifying the old approach to reimbursement instead of developing a new method to pay for twenty-first century healthcare.

Federal reimbursement policy will continue to impede (but not prevent) the evolution of telemedicine until Congress directs otherwise. Short of a statutory dictate to reimburse telemedicine like any

---

TELEMEDICINE IS . . . FREE ON-LINE MEDICAL TEXTBOOKS

Before the Seventh Revolution, the general public was effectively isolated from the wealth of knowledge residing in medical textbooks. Published volumes used to train health professionals were very expensive (usually priced above $100), hard to find (sold in medical bookstores or stored in libraries not readily accessible to the public), and challenging to read (written in arcane professional terms).

These barriers kept outsiders at a distance and reinforced the professional mystique of practitioners, particularly physicians. Few laypeople had the resources, patience, the background, or even the vocabulary to find the information they wanted in medical textbooks, so accessing the knowledge base almost always started with a visit to a doctor.

If knowledge is power, then the telemedicine revolution brought "power to the people" with the Internet launch of emedicine, Inc. in 1998. Absolutely no medical training is necessary to access http://www.emedicine.com, with a home page that reads: "Free online medical textbooks for physicians, veterinarians, medical students, physician assistants, nurse practitioners, nurses and *the public*."

The partners in emedicine, Inc. include Kodak, Genentech, Boston Medical Publishing Corporation, and several large pharmaceutical companies. Not surpris-

other health service—something that is unlikely anytime soon, given a chronic lack of visionary, unifying Congressional leadership on healthcare issues—HCFA reimbursement policy will continue to evolve "behind the curve." Telemedicine will transform healthcare much faster than Medicare will pay for it.

This situation will create many inconveniences for caregivers and patients alike, but both will manage somehow because they have learned to cope with Medicare's roadblocks in the past. Strategies such as gaming the reimbursement system, lobbying to change proposed policies, and appealing final rules have been developed to a fine art over the past few decades. We are saddened by the fact that our nation's largest health plan causes so many resources to be devoted to managing Medicare itself instead of managing the health of its enrollees, but we are confident the industry will survive in spite of it all.

A break in the political logjam probably cannot come any sooner than 2001 for two reasons. First, neither political party wants to yield ground on healthcare issues before the 2000 elections. Second, the Balanced Budget Act of 1997 ties development of telemedicine reimbursement policy to the results of demonstration projects that will not be completed until late in 2001. HCFA is constrained for both of these reasons, so we have some sympathy for its staffers who might like to move at a faster pace.

ingly, their service of free, public access to medical textbooks has attracted a lot of media interest. (See an extensive summation of press coverage under "About Us/Media Releases" on emedicine's Website.) Indeed, this site is seen as an example of a whole new approach to textbook publishing in many fields, not just medicine. (Bronner, E. "For More Textbooks, a Shift from Printed Page to Screen." *The New York Times* (December 1, 1998), A1.)

The on-line textbook in emergency medicine has 665 fully indexed topics, from abdominal trauma to yellow fever, authored by medical school professors and other researchers. Entries include an introduction, review of clinical signs (with numerous photographs, as appropriate), differential diagnosis, workup (lab tests and imaging studies), medications, and follow-up care. Future projects include on-line textbooks for surgery and medicine, dermatology, ophthalmology, neurology, pediatrics and veterinary medicine.

Telemedicine is creating free public access to up-to-date, indexed, searchable, illustrated, and comprehensive medical textbooks . . . imagine the possibilities! Defenders of the old régime will no doubt be appalled, just as kings and priests ultimately came to loathe the arrival of the printing press. But that's what democracy and competition are all about.

Whether they would move forward is uncertain. The overall tone of HCFA's proposed rules to implement BBA-97 suggests the agency has a very limited view of telemedicine—one narrowly focused on using interactive video to make specialty consultations available to Medicare patients in underserved rural areas. In reality, interactive video is only one of several telemedical technologies, specialty consultations constitute only a small portion of all the medical services being revolutionized by telemedicine, and the merger of computers and telecommunications is changing healthcare everywhere from frontier to central city. Indeed, both authors—a longstanding rural resident/farm owner with an extensive background in rural health (Bauer) and a practicing rural family doctor (Ringel)—are annoyed by the implication that telemedicine is a second-best substitute for the "real thing" for rural residents who do not have local access to medical specialists. If telemedicine is good (the authors' clear position), it will be adopted everywhere. If, on the other hand, telemedicine is viewed as a concession made to underserved rural residents, then it should not be adopted anywhere. Neither author sees telemedicine as a rural issue. The sooner it is recognized as a universally potent technology, the better.

We will have more confidence in HCFA when its pronouncements reflect the full scope of telemedicine, suggesting that the staff sees the "big picture" even if Congress does not. In other words, we challenge HCFA to exert some progressive leadership, to become part of the solution rather than the problem.

The first step would be to establish meaningful standards for the medical necessity and effectiveness of all health services. HCFA's foot-dragging on telemedicine reflects a fear that the new technology will foster unnecessary and/or unproductive services and expenses—a dubious and untested assumption which discriminates against telemedicine because HCFA doesn't have any guidelines to validate the medical necessity of face-to-face care, either.[4] Traditional time- and place-dependent medicine is unfairly "grandfathered," to the detriment of telemedicine.

Unnecessary or unproductive care will not be eliminated until uniform standards are developed and applied to all medical services. We believe that telemedicine will fare relatively well when all services are judged by the same criteria. Until then, many useful telemedical services will be uncompensated by Medicare solely because they are new, not because they are wasteful, and many federal dollars will pay for traditional practitioner-patient encounters when telemedicine could have done the same job for less money.

Before addressing the issue of costs, we also urge HCFA to continue rethinking any policies that would direct telemedicine reimbursement to physicians when other practitioners are also qualified to do the work.[5] To be fair, the agency has attempted to reimburse clinical services provided by independent nonphysician practitioners such as nurse practitioners (NPs), physician assistants (PAs), and certified registered nurse anesthetists (CRNAs). However, organized medicine has consistently used its political power to thwart implementation of HCFA's progressive proposals, and the agency is currently being pressured to reimburse telemedical services provided by a nonphysician practitioner only if a physician is present. Reimbursement mechanisms that favor physicians are out-of-touch with the reality of healthcare in the information age because telemedicine is opening the knowledge base of medicine to all practitioners.

Policies that protect traditional medical care are perpetuated by political power, not scientific evidence. Alas, such is the reality of public policy, so politics is the most important key to rationalizing Medicare reimbursement for telemedicine. Research will win a few battles with HCFA, but only political action can win the war with Congress. Final victory will be achieved when Congress is persuaded to tell HCFA to give fair and equal treatment to telemedicine. Telemedicine's proponents must unify and intensify their own political action through active involvement in the American Telemedicine Association (ATA), the Association of Telemedicine Service Providers (ATSP), and other advocacy groups. Above all, consumers must be enlisted to join the ranks because they have the most to gain.

COSTS OF TELEMEDICINE

Policymakers' primary fears of reimbursing unnecessary or second-rate care are followed closely by fears that telemedicine will break the bank. The federal budget has been balanced for the first time in recent memory, so any possible source of increased spending is unwelcome. Telemedicine can expect to face resistance because it has the misfortune of arriving on the scene when the primary (and possibly the only) goal shared across the political spectrum is to avoid deficit spending. Politicians and bureaucrats will not eagerly embrace new domestic programs—including telemedicine—as long as they fear increased spending. Had telemedicine been incorporated into common medical practice just a few years earlier, like minimal access surgery or renal dialysis, Medicare might have started paying for it without much question.

PIONEERS IN TELEMEDICINE: JENNIFER WAYNE-DOPPKE

If creating successful new concepts from diverse experience and varied interests is a common trait among telemedicine's leading developers, then Jennifer Wayne-Doppke is well-qualified for designation as one of the pioneers. A yoga instructor who spent several years training for the Olympics in equestrian events before earning her M.A. in Southwest Asian Studies from the Fletcher School of Law and Diplomacy, she became an expert on the technologies of the Internet. She has worked since the early 1990s as one of the most visible writers, editors, and consultants shaping the development of telemedicine.

Ironically, one of her special qualifications may be her lack of formal training in healthcare. "I see the future of telemedicine primarily through the lens of an experienced Internet observer," she notes, "so I am not limited by memories of healthcare and telemedicine before the Web." Sharing a vision of what lies ahead is her primary goal.

Consequently, she thinks *telemedicine* may already be an outdated term because of its initial association with interactive video and other technologies that are now playing a lesser role in its development. "The word doesn't adequately capture the wide and growing range of possibilities for the future." She prefers to speak in terms of "distributed, technology-enabled health and medical care" but admits this phraseology is a bit too cumbersome to replace telemedicine in everyday use.

Her work on the well-known yearbook, *Healthcare Guide to the Internet,* helped focus attention on the expanding meaning of telemedicine. Subsequent assignment as the first executive editor of the monthly magazine, *Medicine on the Net,* did even more to publicize and popularize the growing role of computer networks in shaping the future of healthcare. A sampling of titles from her articles for *Medicine on the Net* demonstrates the breadth of her vision for telemedicine: "Sharing Files on the Net is as Easy as Zipping, Stuffing, and Crushing," "Test Drive Patient Records on the Web," and "FutureNet: Put the Car on Autopilot, Cruise onto the Internet, Perform Virtual Surgery."

Jennifer Wayne-Doppke has also worked closely with the developers of several other noteworthy publications and Web sites that have moved telemedicine forward. For example, she helped Dr. Tom Ferguson (see pages 76 and 77) do initial research for *The Ferguson Report* and served as a member of the team that launched the well-publicized Website, drkoop.com. More recently, she has been working with onhealth.com, another pioneering venture that is expanding the scope of healthcare by bringing together patients and practitioners and expanding the useful information available to both.

Her work is motivated by a strong belief that our healthcare delivery system is improved by the flow of accurate and timely information to all parties. More direct care, too, will occur over the Net. "Ideally, telemedicine will provide high-quality, comprehensive services to populations and geographic areas that have not had full access in the past. It will enable more patient participation and extend the reach of our country's leading provider organizations." However, she believes that a few years will be needed for public policy and reimbursement to recognize the true benefits of telemedicine.

Ms. Wayne-Doppke sees telemedicine as a tool for "medicine at its best." Her vision of distributed, technology-enabled healthcare includes doctors who write information prescriptions and multimedia platforms that will allow many high-tech services—including surgery—to be provided in patients' homes instead of hospitals. She expects that all the media comprising telemedicine today will blend in the not-too-distant future.

"The limiting factors are bandwidth and infrastructure," she believes. She is correspondingly surprised that the giant corporate producers of bandwidth and infrastructure have not taken a more active role in developing products specifically for telemedicine. In her view, the growth of telemedicine will really take off when large manufacturers choose to push the healthcare potential of their software and hardware. "When the Fortune 500 companies decide to move, watch out," she says of the potential for explosive growth. Jennifer also believes that cable networks, not telephone lines, could ultimately become the dominant backbone of the system.

Last, and definitely not least, consumers are a very powerful and positive force in her vision of the future. "The consumer-driven quest for better health information will determine much of what will happen," she believes. She thinks doctors overall are slow to recognize and respect consumers' powerful role in shaping the future of healthcare in general and telemedicine in particular, but she has enormous respect for the doctors who "get it" and thinks they will have no trouble staying very busy in the future.

But isn't leadership in developing consumer-oriented Websites inconsistent with her graduate study of Asian trade routes and cultural interactions? "Not at all," she replies, "if you think of the Internet as a trade route and E-commerce as the Silk Road of the twenty-first century."

Caregivers are also free to engage in telemedicine across state lines, as long as they are licensed in the state where the patient is located.

This approach is intended to protect the patient by conferring a right to hold practitioners liable to the professional practice standards of the state in which the patient receives the care (which is presumably the patient's state of residence). Seen from a jurisdictional perspective, a patient can sue allegedly negligent practitioners in the appropriate court of the patient's state of residence. The legal foundation of this arrangement made more sense in the past when standards of practice were local. Today, patients are effectively protected by national standards of care that are largely promulgated and disseminated by electronic means.

Practitioners in some states are even beginning to demand protection from out-of-state practitioners because telemedicine creates a national market. In response to intense political pressure from state medical societies, a small number of states have recently passed laws to hinder or prevent interstate telemedicine. We believe the motives behind this recent movement are purely anti-competitive, and we do not expect such protectionist legislation to survive for very long. Consumers and courts have different, pro-competitive ideas.

The mismatch between today's technology and state practice acts derives from the historical fact that states have always licensed health professionals. The federal government rejected the idea of licensing professionals back during the period of Jacksonian democracy in the mid-nineteenth century, and states have retained this power ever since. Consequently, caregivers who practice in more than one state, such as those who work in multistate metropolitan areas like Kansas City or Philadelphia, have always obtained licenses in the two or three states where they might see a patient.

Telemedicine creates the possibility that the patient can be anywhere in the country.[9] Getting fifty state licenses is extraordinarily difficult, if not impossible. (However, we have met a few radiologists and other consulting physicians with licenses in as many as forty states.) Creating a national license for telemedicine is one possible solution to the problem, and it might happen within a decade or two. Political activity to promote telemedicine at the federal level is extremely important and should be supported by all who are committed to the Seventh Revolution, but the current political climate in Washington suggests that progress will most likely be made on other fronts first.

Three different and promising solutions are already in fairly advanced stages of development.

- The creation of a *multistate compact* to authorize telenursing across the lines of participating states is being pursued under leadership of the National Council of State Boards of Nursing.[10] As a practical alternative to establishing a common, identical license (the general theory behind a federal solution), the compact model applies the concept of reciprocity. States that pass legislation to join a compact would agree to recognize nursing licenses granted by all other states that join the same telenursing compact (somewhat like the way states agree to recognize tourists' drivers licenses without establishing identical requirements for being licensed as a driver). Nursing representatives in more than a dozen states are already working with their state legislatures to authorize reciprocal recognition of nursing licenses under a multistate compact, and some success is expected soon. (Utah has already passed a law to authorize participation in a multistate compact for telenursing.) Compacts will not immediately create a national solution, but they would be a very big step in the right direction.

- A plan to allow interstate telemedicine based on a *model state practice act limited to telemedicine* is being developed by the Federation of State Medical Boards.[11] Under this approach, states would create a special license to regulate the practice of telemedicine across state lines, that is, a license conferring only defined privileges of telemedicine. Practitioners who wished to use telemedicine to treat a patient in a state where they do not have a regular license would be required to get the other state's license limited to the practice of telemedicine. The model act defines common rules for medical records and patient confidentiality, in addition to stringent requirements for maintaining full licensure in a participating state. Requirements for professional board certification and continuing professional education could also be included.

- Another approach is *licensing Internet practice sites*. This model, being developed by the National Association of State Boards of Pharmacy,[12] establishes minimum standards for verifying that Internet pharmacies and their personnel are licensed in good standing with the appropriate state board(s) of pharmacy and other regulatory bodies. Internet pharmacies can apply for certification under the Verified Internet Pharmacy Practice Sites (VIPPS) program and then display the VIPPS logo on their Web pages. Consumers will be able to use the designation to distinguish between on-line pharmacies that adhere to state laws and those that may not. Several entrepreneurs have operated "fly by night" pharmacy sites on the Web, so site licensing by legitimate professional organizations could be a very important key to the future success of telemedicine.

As implied by discussion of the VIPPS model, some telemedical practices will undoubtedly develop in gray areas of the law, and a few providers will openly violate established laws of licensure. Statutes and case law will be challenged to keep up with the practices made possible by the Seventh Revolution. Telemedicine's ethical advocates must maintain a high level of political involvement in order to ensure that telemedicine manages itself in the interests of consumer protection. To that end, the new licensing processes must be understandable and visible to consumers.

SECURITY AND PRIVACY

Telemedicine sometimes gets a bum rap when the discussion turns to protecting privacy. People have good reason to be concerned about breaches in the confidentiality of their medical records, but many wrongly assume that an electronic record is less secure than a traditional paper record. Such concerns were perfectly legitimate when

---

TELEMEDICINE IS . . . COMMUNITY HEALTH INFORMATION

Healthcare discussions often overlook the fact that some medical services are provided to the community, not to individuals. Public health is even defined as population medicine. Its services, such as sanitation and prevention programs, affect individuals' health even though they are not provided in doctors' offices or hospitals. Just as a general analysis of healthcare should encompass public health (which, sadly, is often not the case), a focused inquiry into telemedicine must consider community health.

How might telemedicine liberate public health professionals from the constraints of space and time and improve the efficiency and effectiveness of activities like publicizing existing health resources and establishing new programs? One innovative answer to this important question is the Community Tool Box (http://ctb.lsi.ukans.edu.ctb/).

A Website created and maintained by the University of Kansas Work Group on Health Promotion and Community Development (Lawrence, Kansas) and AHEC/Community Partners (Amherst, Massachusetts), the Community Tool Box

telemedicine arrived on the scene, but thanks to recent developments in on-line security, electronic information can be protected much better than paper records.

- *Authentication* is becoming a first-line standard in the protection of electronic information in telemedicine networks. For years, anyone who has accessed an electronic file over the Internet has been identified by user name and password, but lapses could easily occur through unauthorized uses, such as a stolen password. Now, commercial-off-the-shelf (COTS) devices can be used to compare a fingerprint, retinal scan, or voice print with a file copy to verify that the on-line person is truly the person he or she claims to be. Websites and computers can also be given verifiable and traceable identifying marks. With these protections, telemedical records can be made much more secure than information on paper. The exact identity of a person perusing a paper record is seldom ascertained or recorded, but electronic systems can keep complete records of each individual who accessed information. They can also create an audit trail that tracks all modifications made to the record, an important protection that is practically impossible to provide in a paper records system.

- *Authorization* is the second mechanism that can provide telemedicine with greater levels of security than those found in traditional healthcare. System software can make sure that

gives free and immediate access to lots of new ideas, related materials, discussions with experienced peers, and other helpful resources that have previously required a trip to the library or attendance at a conference. And you don't have to be a health professional to use it, which means more people can get involved.

This growing site currently has 135 virtual "how to" tools that can be used to conduct a needs assessment, write a grant, prepare a public information campaign, solve problems, evaluate a program, create a change-oriented environment, train leaders and volunteers, or perform many other community-oriented tasks. It hosts ongoing electronic forums to facilitate discussion between people working on the same problems all over the country (even the world).

It also fulfills the other requirements of our definition of telemedicine by producing empowerment, information, choice, and competition. Thanks to the Tool Box, any community-oriented person can now learn about different ways to meet public health needs without paying for consultants or conferences—which leaves more to spend directly on community health. That's at least a little bit revolutionary.

the authenticated person who is seeking electronic information is authorized to see it. In addition, electronic records can easily be segmented so that access is limited to certain types of information. For example, the list of a patient's prescription medications, often a clue to physical or mental conditions a patient prefers to keep private, can be kept off-limits to a radiology technologist who only needs to see information relevant to taking an X ray. In comparison, traditional paper records are almost always kept together in a single folder, readily accessible to prying eyes that want to see more than they should.

- *Encryption* is a protection that can now be built into telemedicine systems. An encryption algorithm works somewhat like a paper shredder when information is fed into it, but it can quickly reassemble the pieces at the other end of the line for someone who is authorized to view the information. Encryption software uses a mathematical function to scramble information so that it is completely unintelligible to anyone who does not have the numerical key to decode it. Only authorized users can unscramble the data. Paper records are, of course, readable to anyone who gets access to them at any time (which means they can also be photocopied and disseminated outside the system). Providers of telemedicine services can now include encryption capabilities in their systems with relative ease and little cost. Even if information gets into the wrong hands, it is meaningless when properly encrypted. Paper-based systems offer no such protection.

Security systems for telemedicine can be made even more powerful through the use of dedicated communications lines and network access controls (called firewalls). Effective combinations of hardware and software can be used to provide desired levels of security, so clinicians or managers responsible for implementing telemedicine can approach the task with the assurance that protecting confidentiality is now a whole lot easier than it was just a few years ago. Information security always will be a problem, but it can be addressed very effectively in the electronic realm of telemedicine by the savvy use of ubiquitous technologies.

No information system will ever be perfect. However, electronic health information systems can be made more secure than traditional records, and they can provide some protections that are not found in paper systems (e.g., records of all users and data modifications). Given these recent improvements in electronic security, two far more difficult challenges related to privacy are health professionals' use of cellular telephones (which are easily intercepted) and implementation of the Health Insurance Portability and Accountability Act of 1996—a flawed federal law that may seriously complicate the transmission of healthcare data in all forms.

QUALITY AND GUIDELINES

Last, but not least, telemedicine will rightly be held accountable for the quality of services that are delivered across the barriers of time and place. Quality has been defined and judged from several different perspectives over the years. A three-tier analysis based on the works of Professor Avedis Donabedian (University of Michigan) prevailed from the 1960s through the early 1980s. It judged quality on the basis of the structure of the delivery system (e.g., whether a hospital had the appropriate equipment to deliver a particular service), the process of care (e.g., the extent to which different personnel worked together according to specified standards), and outcomes (e.g., patients' post-treatment conditions compared with expected norms). Accreditation by national organizations such as the Joint Commission for the Accreditation of Healthcare Organizations (JCAHO) gained considerable strength as a proxy for quality over the same period.

Several additional concepts of quality came into use in the 1980s. In particular, outcomes measurement moved from internal assessments based on expected performance to external comparisons with all like providers in a market area. Various groups began not only to issue "report cards," but to post the grades for all to see. For example, government agencies and purchaser coalitions published data that compared cardiac surgeons' survival rates and hospitals' deviations from expected mortality. Many observers (the present authors included) have raised serious questions about the validity of such comparisons in the absence of consistent and meaningful methods to adjust for differences in patients' initial conditions. Safety, appropriateness, and consumer satisfaction have also been used as measures of quality.

However, the important point for purposes of this analysis is that, by the early 1990s, quality assessment had moved from an internal review—one where accreditation status was usually the only quality indicator released to the public—to a very open process where numerous performance indicators were published in the newspaper or reported on the evening news. The shift from closed to open quality assessment was fully operationalized with the formation of the National Council

PIONEERS IN TELEMEDICINE: PAUL ZIMNIK, D.O.

Unlike many health professionals who entered the realm of telemedicine in mid-career by accident, Paul Zimnik was the right age to grow with it from the beginning by choice. After riding the early waves of computer-based education and electronic games as a high school student on Florida's Gulf coast in the 1970s, he headed to California for a degree in computer science.

Undergraduate studies at California Polytechnic State University put him in the right place at the right time. Many of his classmates and instructors were moonlighting with start-up companies in nearby Silicon Valley at the time of the area's most explosive growth, and Paul became involved in several leading-edge development projects. Most significantly, he had the opportunity to work directly with Steve Jobs on the development of Apple's Macintosh—ultimately marketed as "the computer for the rest of us."

He then pursued medical training at the Kirksville College of Osteopathic Medicine, fulfilling a lifelong dream to become a doctor. The dream began in junior high school when he was exposed to the patient-focused concepts of Dr. Andrew Still, founder of both the osteopathic alternative to allopathic medicine and the Kirksville College. Dr. Zimnik's decision to become an osteopathic physician was also consistent with a general philosophical belief in the principle of self-determination.

The sense of individual empowerment embodied in Still's writings and Jobs' products reinforced Zimnik's decision to become a doctor who would use computers to involve patients in their own healthcare. Dr. Zimnik pursued his medical training with a belief that networked computers would change the relationship between doctors and patients just as powerfully as desktop computers were liberating employees and customers from the tyranny of the mainframe. His infectious enthusiasm for the future of telemedicine is rooted in a longstanding belief that it is the foundation of a global, consumer-centric, market-driven healthcare system.

Military service provided the perfect environment for Dr. Zimnik to put his ideas into practice. He joined the U.S. Air Force upon graduation from medical school in 1988 and began the residency program in psychiatry at Wright-Patterson AFB in Dayton, Ohio. For reasons detailed in Chapter 6, telemedicine was adopted as a major solution to problems posed by the military's new political and economic realities, so Capt. Zimnik was soon assigned to direct many development projects at the military's telemedicine command at Ft. Dietrick, Maryland. Having completed his military service obligation in mid-1998, he continues his leadership as a consultant to numerous telemedicine projects in the United States and other countries.

Dr. Zimnik has always held a broad view of telemedicine, one that goes far beyond the concept's initial identification with interactive video. He prefers to talk of digital medicine because this terminology focuses attention on distributing digitized information rather than overcoming distance. Indeed, he has placed considerable emphasis on digital acquisition, storage, and transmission of all health information as part of his leadership at TATRC. Analog technologies are definitely not part of his long-range vision.

He is committed to continued evolution and leadership in the direction of informed, self-directed care. "Every time we ask ourselves which path to take, we'll make the right choice as long as we choose the path that empowers the individual consumer." He is definitely not the type of doctor who wants to protect the traditional one-way relationship between submissive patient and paternalistic physician, and he recognizes the threat that telemedicine represents to doctors who are comfortable with the past.

Dr. Zimnik also perceives telemedicine as a force inevitably moving our health system toward decentralization, organizationally as well as clinically. "Large systems and big buildings are totally contrary to the future of healthcare and totally inconsistent with its distributed future," he argues. "Practitioners will become differentiated in the process of decentralization. Some will work directly with patients, while others will provide the care team with virtual support. Some of the most effective care will be delivered by practitioners who never meet patients face-to-face."

In spite of his international recognition as a pioneer in the development of telemedicine, he does not feel that he is "steering the ship." Rather, he believes that the technological revolution itself is the driving force. "The future will be the same regardless of the individuals who become leaders. Progress will occur because the technologies—not the leaders—compel it to happen."

Long interested in Oriental philosophy, Dr. Zimnik has developed a tsunami analogy to summarize this view of the inevitability of the coming changes in healthcare. "Telemedicine's leaders have done nothing more that recognize the power of a 300-foot wave that has already been generated by forces beyond their control. The revolution will occur because of this naturally occurring wave; the leaders did not create the wave."

on Quality Assurance (NCQA), a purchaser consortium that issues comparative reports on how well health plans and providers comply with procedures that presumably measure best practices.

Medical journals and trade publications have recently published articles that question the effectiveness of report cards issued by (or on behalf of) government agencies and employers that purchase health plans. The information is not obviously useful or understandable to very many consumers. Telemedicine largely makes this issue irrelevant because empowered consumers can now use the Internet to share quality assessments in terms that really matter to them. For example, NCQA bases its quality assessments on criteria like the percentage of at-risk females who receive mammograms or the relative number of diabetics who receive nutrition counseling. You can bet that consumers will care at least as much, if not more, about difficulties in getting appointments or their practitioners' ability to answer questions in layperson's language. Chat rooms, on-line support groups, and E-mail distribution lists of people with specific interests (called listservs) provide a forum for consumers interested in sharing information. All these Internet-based mechanisms will become quickly familiar to people who use telemedicine. (For example, eBay is an on-line auction which maintains an ongoing forum where buyers rate the goods and services they buy. This model will undoubtedly grow in the healthcare marketplace.)

Consumers and purchasers will certainly benefit from having access to both sorts of information (e.g., objective report cards and subjective consumer comments).[13] Of course, the quality and usefulness of information found in a consumer chat room will be challenged by the same commentators who raise questions about professional report cards, and many of their concerns will be valid. However, practitioners and health systems will not be able to throw the baby out with the bath water. The Internet is here to stay, and it will be a very powerful contributor to the consumer empowerment made possible by telemedicine. Progressive providers will rise to the challenge, learn to understand their customers, and develop new professional skills to help consumers get better healthcare. Providers who resist the new, electronic dimension of quality will be lucky to survive very far into the twenty-first century.

Finally, one of the most important advances in quality assessment has been the development and use of clinical practice guidelines (CPGs) over the past decade. CPGs are roughly equivalent to the checklists pilots use to ensure that they do the right things at the right time when flying an airplane.[14] In healthcare, guideline development usually begins with a panel of experts who review the published literature on different ways to treat a condition and to identify clinical interventions that produce desired outcomes. The members of the expert panel then develop a consensus position on steps that need to be taken to maximize the possibilities of producing desired outcomes. Day-to-day delivery of care can be guided by the specific instructions in the CPG.

A specific example is undoubtedly better than an academic discussion of quality guidelines applied to telemedicine. Therefore, we close this chapter with actual guidelines for providing home care by telemedicine, as approved in 1999 by the American Telemedicine Association's Special Interest Group on Telehome Care. The ATA homecare guidelines provide a good, comprehensive model for other groups to follow in their own efforts to promote high-quality telemedical services.

ATA TELE-HOMECARE CLINICAL GUIDELINES

PATIENT CRITERIA

- Informed written consent must be obtained from the patient or designee before beginning the use of video visits and should be a part of the plan of care and in the clinical record.

- During the initial visit, an assessment should be conducted to determine the access to utilities and safety concerns appropriate for equipment installation.

- The patient may un-enroll from tele-homecare at any time without fear of retribution (loss of home health agency services).

- Patients (or their designated caregiver) must demonstrate the ability to use and maintain the equipment according to agency policy.

- Patients who require interpreters must be so identified, and agency policy and procedures to deal with language barriers must be followed to ensure that these patients are not discriminated against.

- Patients or their designees who cannot demonstrate the ability to operate the equipment appropriately, and for whom translation is not available, should be excluded form tele-homecare.

- Patients need to be trained and provided written information in their homes regarding procedures to operate and maintain equipment. Such information may include diagrams to ensure patients are placing equipment, i.e. placement of a stethoscope, on the appropriate part of the body.

- Patients cannot be viewed through the video without their knowledge or prior written consent. If other agency personnel or visitors come into viewing site,

ATA Tele-Homecare Clinical Guidelines Continued

the patient must be made aware of their presence, and patient's approval
must be obtained for such personnel to participate in the video visit. If a third
remote site is participating in the video visit the patient must again be aware
and approve of such participation.

- Patient satisfaction regarding video visits should be a part of CQI protocols.
- The first and last home visit should be done in-person and not through a video
  visit.

HEALTH PROVIDER CRITERIA

- A home healthcare agency may provide tele-homecare visits to accomplish
  and/or to enhance patient care under circumstances when "hands-on care" is
  not required.
- A physician order to integrate tele-homecare into the plan of care must be obtained.
- Video visits may be provided by RNs, social workers, LPNs, physical therapists, speech therapists, occupational therapists, nutritionists, physicians and/
  or nurse practitioners, or others within the scope of practice for that category
  of practitioner.
- The agency personnel providing tele-homecare must document each video visit
  in the patient's chart.
- All tele-homecare providers as listed under bullet #3 above must be trained
  and demonstrate the ability to do video visits on the technology being used by
  the agency.
- In case of equipment failure an in-person visit should be scheduled as soon as
  possible to ensure adherence to the plan of care.
- The staff should demonstrate the ability to correctly use the technology and
  troubleshoot common problems. They should also have written troubleshooting
  guidelines to follow and a method for follow-up if problems are not quickly resolved.
- Each state will decide if they will allow "across state line video visits".
- Changes in video visit frequency will be treated like changes in other parts of
  the plan of treatment and should be approved by the physician.
- Agencies must provide clearly written information to patients regarding use of
  the equipment, in addition to in-person training provided at the onset of tele-
  homecare.
- Patients must be given clear written instructions as to who to call in case
  problems arise. Patients need to be regularly informed in writing of the difference between using tele-homecare and an emergency medical response system
  to avoid a potential delay in need for "911" emergency care.

ATA Tele-Homecare Clinical Guidelines Concluded

- Agencies should provide a plan of action to provide unscheduled video visits (supervisors or other staff in the office should be available if the patient case manager is absent).
- Video visits may be incorporated into critical pathways.
- If 24-hour tele-homecare service is available, agencies must provide written instructions to patients for contact after-hours with care providers.
- After-hours video visit coverage could be accomplished by on-call or after hours staff, call center staff, or emergency room staff. Arrangements for this application could be done through a remote, central location.

TECHNOLOGY CRITERIA

- The technology used should be based on the patient's clinical and functional needs. Based upon the clinical needs of the patient many components may be included such as; two way interactive video, telephonic stethoscope, blood pressure and pulse. Other optional equipment may include oximetry, EKG, glucose meter, other medical devices, Internet capabilities, etc.
- The equipment based at the central station should include a log-in code and password to maintain patient privacy and record security.
- Upon installation, the tele-homecare equipment should be checked for accuracy against standard devices.
- Procedures must be written and in place to clean and maintain equipment (per agency health and safety codes and infection control standards) at installation, while in the patient's home, and on return to agency.
- Installation kits should be made with written instructions for the staff and should include supplies needed to ensure best picture quality, e.g., small table lamp if necessary and extension cords. Supplies will be distributed according to site and technology chosen.
- Safety instructions should be given to patients and reviewed at installation and future times as necessary.
- Instructions on whom to call for patient questions and concerns regarding equipment must be provided to patients and agency staff.

NOTES

1. For helpful assistance in finding and comparing state-level laws, legal rulings, and administrative regulations concerning telemedicine, consult two publications of Legamed, Inc., *1999 Compendium of Telemedicine Laws: Selected Statute Excerpts*

and Article Citations Relating to Telemedicine, and *Telemedlaw,* a quarterly review of recent developments in telemedicine. Additional information is available at www.legamed.com.

2. For a more detailed and well-referenced historical review of underlying issues, see Grigsby, J and JH Sanders. "Telemedicine: Where It Is and Where It's Going," *Annals of Internal Medicine* 129(2): 123–127 (July 15, 1998).

3. "Medicare Program: Payment for Teleconsultation in Rural Health Professional Shortage Areas," *Federal Register* 63(119): Proposed Rules 33884 (June 22, 1998).

4. The National Institutes of Health, most notably through the Agency for Health Care Policy and Research (AHCPR), have taken some progressive initial steps toward developing the science of health services research, but much remains to be done. Visit http://www.ahcpr.gov to review the agency's work.

5. *Not What the Doctor Ordered,* op. cit., explores this issue in depth.

6. Cost-effectiveness analysis is an economic tool for comparing the costs of different ways of producing a specific output. The least-expensive method for producing a desired result is the most cost-effective. It is often confused with a different concept, cost-benefit analysis, which ranks different investments in terms of the total value of benefits yielded over time per dollar of expenditure.

7. For an example of Web-based marketing surveys, see Gillespie, G. "But Are They Satisfied?" *Health Data Management* (May 1999): 90–92.

8. For a more detailed review of differences between state laws, see Siwicki, B. "Telemedicine Providers' Progress Impeded at the Border," *Health Data Management* (May 1999): 94–102.

9. Obviously, telemedicine can also be delivered across national borders. For example, one of the world's best known gurus, a direct spiritual descendant of the mahatma, recently decided to give American telemedicine a try. He submitted digital pictures of the soles of his feet, made thick by years of walking barefooted. He answered an on-line health questionnaire, indicating that he was frequently weak because he ate a meager vegetarian diet and suffered from bad breath because he did not brush his teeth. The electronic system evaluated his information and issued a preliminary diagnosis within seconds—a super calloused fragile

mystic plagued with halitosis.

10. http://www.ncsbn.org
11. http://www.fsmb.org
12. http://www.nabp.net
13. For a good example of an on-line resource that nicely blends different types of quality information so that purchasers and consumers can make fully informed choices, visit the Website of the Greater Detroit Area Health Council, Inc., http://www.gdahc.org. Two subsections of this site, the Health Plan Navigator (/hpn) and the Health Information Action Group (/hiag), demonstrate the promising possibilities for establishing multidimensional databases on quality.
14. See http://www.guidelines.gov for current examples of guidelines that have passed a professional review process.

8

C H A P T E R

Annotated References

In today's fast-paced world, the phrase "setting it down on paper" sounds almost as archaic as "carving it in stone" once did. Information ages at an alarming rate. The more permanent the storage medium, the longer the imprinted information may outlast its usefulness. (Perhaps published information should be dated, like food: "Best if used by . . . ")

As authors, we knew before we wrote one word of this book that significant portions would be out-of-date on the day it was printed. Still, books are wonderful, portable, analog devices for transmitting large amounts of information in a coherent whole to a targeted audience (those who would buy or borrow the book). Books as a medium won't disappear, but they will change with the times.

Two characteristics of this project will, we hope, prolong the shelf life of our work. First, we have taken a broad view, which should give readers a correspondingly long-run perspective. The second "preservative" is this chapter, which points the way to many useful information sources. In keeping with the subject and the times, the majority of the entries in the following list include the URLs (Universal Resource Locators) of helpful Websites. Since they exist in the virtual world of electronic space, you can expect these sites to evolve rapidly (or cease to exist) and to interconnect and point beyond themselves in ever richer and more useful ways.

So, reader, when you venture out beyond the boundaries of this book, you can start at a likely-sounding site from this reference list and "surf" your way into all sorts of fascinating places to update your knowledge on topics in telemedicine or, ultimately, anything else available on the Web. You are free to create your very own road map for navigating the future of healthcare.

We researched and wrote this book in a Web-enabled way, sometimes pursuing information directly and at other times browsing to see where we might be taken by our instincts, curiosity, and luck. Though we used the Internet to track down information, we also relied extensively on interviews, books, journals, and newspapers. Each of us organized the resulting heaps of analog and digital information in his own idiosyncratic way, consistent with our personal experiences, styles, and visions of telemedicine.

Assuming this book inspires you to strike off on your own to learn more about telemedicine, how do you find what you really want to know? And, once you've found it, how do you know whether you can trust it? These questions are the theme for yet another full-length book. Knowing that you don't want a two hundred page appendix to this one, we will instead endeavor briefly to present a very practical introductory approach to dealing with the quantity and assessing the quality of information available on-line.

Branding is a good place to start. If the information is posted by a federal agency (e.g. NIH, NLM, AHCPR), a respected university or medical center, a reputable doctor or researcher, or a well-established professional association (e.g. IEEE, NIST, ISO), it is probably pretty reliable. "Reliable" does not necessarily mean "true," since all information, especially scientific, is subject to change as knowledge progresses. "Reliable" means merely the best information available for now—information supported by professional consensus.

Information that is supplied by somebody who is selling something—from pharmaceutical manufacturer to technology vendor—should be viewed more skeptically. There are some commercial Websites where you might consider rolling up your pant legs before stepping in. Of course, any information—no matter how good the brand—needs to be evaluated critically. Deciding how critical to be at each step on an information journey will help you to weigh automatically the value of what you pick up on your quest. Always keep the source in mind. The process is quite similar to what you go through to evaluate any other source of information. Skepticism is key.

All sorts of schemes are in the works for rating content, none of them able to match the exponential growth rate of Websites and their interconnections. Healthweb, which contains a set of links selected by librarians, is one site for encountering information sources with a stamp of quality. Medsite is another.

Recently an outfit called "Health on the Net" (HON) has been lending its imprimatur to medical sites. Adherents to the HON code agree to a set of principles including: relying on health professionals as information sources; striving to support, not replace, the doctor-patient relationship; guaranteeing the confidentiality of users; providing links, balanced evidence, and contact information; and being forthright about commercial support.

Weighing information is still a very human activity, hard to delegate and not likely to be automated soon. Indeed, both authors believe that all users should devote more attention than ever to evaluating the quality of information, now that technology allows us to find it with less effort.

You can control the amount of stuff you have to plow through in order to get what you want. To prevent being inundated with information you don't want or need, be very stingy about giving out personal information, including your E-mail address. Because E-mail can be sent as easily to ten million as to ten—there are no pages to fold, no stamps to lick—junk E-mail can clutter your computer's mailbox faster than fourth class "snail mail" can overflow your mailbox at home. Give your address only to people and places from whom you really want to hear.

If you belong to one of the mega-Internet service providers such as AOL, you may find that you are the target of tons of unsolicited junk E-mail. E-mail programs do have filters that can be set up to discard unopened mail from certain sources or with certain characteristics that smell like junk. If you feel you're losing the war, switch to a small, local ISP that probably hasn't caught the attention of many electronic junk mailers.

When you embark on a search, use one of the established and recognized search engines: Excite, Lycos, Yahoo, HotBot, etc. Determine which ones you like because all use different approaches to looking for information. Most of them have options for doing searches, which, though called "advanced," are fairly easy to use. They employ simple concepts from Boolean algebra, allowing you to include and exclude terms that narrow or broaden a search until you get what you are really seeking. Learning to use the advanced features of one or more search engines so you can improve the efficiency of your searches is worth the effort.

Once you've found the information you want, check out the hotlinks (i.e., the connections to related sites). Now you're surfing, going

from site to site, seeing where the connections lead you. Plan on getting lost, finding yourself some place very far removed from where you
started out and not at all clear about how you got there.

Every Web browser has bookmarks that will take you directly
back to any site you have marked. Well-organized bookmark folders,
which can be classified and subclassified, can keep you in touch with
any place on the Web, always at *your* initiative. Learn how to use this
function if you are not familiar with it. You can always create bookmarks to track your path through the information thicket. Other ex-
ceptionally useful navigation aids include your browser's "back" button
which will retrace your steps one at a time and the history folder
which contains a complete list of where you have just been.

The Internet is seductive. People "lose" hours and days surfing. If
you have the time, there's nothing wrong with that. Browsing in this
hyper-linked world, you are likely to uncover some interesting and
even some useful stuff. If you don't have the time to burn, set a time
limit before you embark. If you don't find what you need, ask an expert
for help or try again later.

Remember librarians. Their jobs have changed dramatically in
the information age. Librarians are much more than keepers of the
archives and defenders of the Dewey decimal system. They are experts
at helping people to track down, weigh, and interpret information—
and they are generally quite skilled in conducting electronic searches.

Trust yourself. If you have heretofore lived in an intellectual
world populated by books and journals, you have already developed
critical skills for finding and evaluating information. The Internet is
just another way of organizing and presenting information—one with
lots of glitz, hype, and promise. Plan on stumbling around for awhile.
You will learn eventually to access a mind-boggling array of resources
right from your desktop. Ultimately, you control what information you
get and, most importantly, what it means.

The following list is truly a drop in the information ocean. Entries
were chosen either because they are mentioned in the text or because,
in the authors' experience, they are good launch points. From the moment you click on your first hyperlink, you will be on your own, unique
voyage as an active participant in the telemedicine revolution.

- *Access to Medical Informatics for Continuing Medical
  Education,* 2nd ed.: *A Basic Guide to Access of Medical
  Information via Print and Electronic Media*
  A primer for using telemedicine and other electronic means
  for CME.

Alliance for Continuing Medical Education
1025 Montgomery Hwy., Suite 208
Birmingham, AL 35216
phone: 205-824-1355
fax: 205-824-1357
Web: *www.acme-assn.org*

- *Accessing Medical Information from a Desert Island with Telephone Service: How to Get and Organize the Information You Need to Practice Most Effectively*
Dated regarding electronic medical resources but comprehensive and practical in its overall approach to meeting clinicians' needs for medical information.
  by Marc Ringel
  Greeley, Co.: Desert Island Press, 1993 and 1995
  E-mail: *mringel@lhsnet.org*

- ACR-NEMA   See American College of Radiology and the National Equipment Manufacturers' Association.

- American College of Radiology and the National Equipment Manufacturers' Association (ACR-NEMA)

ACR	NEMA
1891 Preston White Dr.	1300 N. 17th St.
Reston, VA 20191	Rosslyn, VA 22209
phone: 703-648-8900	phone: 703-841-3285
fax: 703-391-0391	fax: 703-841-3385
Web: *www.acr.org*	Web: *http://www.nema.org*

- American Medical Association
  515 State St.
  Chicago, IL 60610
  phone: 312-464-5000
  fax: 303-486-4740
  Web: *http://www.ama-assn.org*
  CME Locator:
  http://www.ama-org/med-sci/cme/cme.htm

- American Medical Informatics Association (AMIA)
Devoted to promotion development and application of medical informatics to patient care.
  4915 St. Elmo Ave., Suite 401
  Bethesda, MD 20814
  phone: 301-657-1291
  fax: 301-657-1296
  Web: *www.amia.org*

- American National Standards Institute (ANSI)
    11 W. 42nd St.
    New York, NY 10036
    phone: 212-642-8904
    fax: 212-398-0023
    Web: *www.ansi.org*
- American Telemedicine Association
  Information clearinghouse, involved in developing
  standards.
    1010 Vermont Ave., N.W., Suite 301
    Washington, DC 20005
    phone: 202-628-4700
    fax: 202-628-4277
    Web: *http://www.atmeda.org*
- AMIA   See American Medical Informatics Association.
- ANSI   See American National Standards Institute.
- Apple Computer, Inc.
    1 Infinite Loop
    Cupertino, CA 95014
    phone: 408-996-1010
    Web: *www.apple.com*
- Association of Telemedicine Service Providers (ATSP)
    7276 SW Beaverton-Hillsdale Hwy., Suite 400
    Portland, OR 97225
    phone: 503-222-2406
    fax: 503-223-7581
    Web: *http://www.atsp.org*
- ATSP   See Association of Telemedicine Service Providers.
- Blue Shield of California
    Web: *www.blueshieldca.com*
- Centers for Disease Control
  The U.S. Centers for Disease Control and Prevention is the
  foremost public health agency and research organization in
  the country. Their Website is filled with information for
  laypeople and professionals, including advice for travelers to
  foreign countries.
    Web: *http://www.cdc.gov/*
- CHESS   See Comprehensive Health Enhancement Support
  System.

- Community of Science, Inc.
A network of scientists and researchers dedicated to connecting collaborators and research opportunities. Keyword searches (e.g. "telemedicine") yield a list of grants and colleagues.
    Web: *http://www.cos.com/*
- Community Tool Box
A Website that is chock full of tools for assessing and affecting health from a community perspective. (See "Telemedicine is . . . community health information," pages 170 and 171.)
    Web: *http://ctb.lsi.ukans.edu/ctb/*
- Comprehensive Health Enhancement Support System (CHESS)
A computer-based patient and family support system. (See "Telemedicine is . . . empowered patients," pages 116 and 117.)
    CHESS Research Consortium
    Room 1109 WARF Building, 610 Walnut Street
    Madison, WI 53705
    phone: 608-262-4746
    Web: *www.harthosp.org/Chess/chess.htm*
- *Computer: A History of the Information Machine*
Well-done history of the electronics revolution.
    by Martin Campbell-Kelly and William Aspray
    New York: Basic Books, Collins Publishers, 1996
- *The Computer-Based Medical Record: An Essential Technology for Health Care,* rev. ed.
The Institute of Medicine's blueprint for the computerized patient record.
    by Richard S. Dick, Elaine B. Steen, Don E. Detmer, eds.
    Washington, D.C.: National Academy Press, 1997
- The Computer-based Patient Record Institute (CPRI)
    Web: *http://www.cpri.org/*
- CPRI   See The Computer-based Patient Record Institute.
- *Demanding Medical Excellence: Doctors and Accountability in the Information Age*
A broad and deep look at how information systems are changing the nature of medical practice.
    by Michael L. Millenson
    Chicago: University of Chicago Press, 1997

- Department of Defense Telemedicine
  A good staging area for exploring the DOD's extensive work
  on telemedicine. Links to many civilian sites.
     Web: *http://www.tatrc.org/*
- Department of Health and Human Services
  This site has information for patients and links to a wide
  swath of federal health organizations.
     Web: *http://www.os.dhhs.gov*
- DICOM   See Digital Image and Communications in Medicine.
- Digital Image and Communications in Medicine (DICOM)
     Web: *http://rpiwww.mdacc.tmc.edu/~jrus-sell/dicoms*
- Doctor Koop's Community
  A myriad of information written for the consumer on diseases,
  tests, surgery, health, and wellness. Named for its founder, the
  famous Reagan Administration Surgeon General, Dr. C.
  Everett Koop.
     Web: *http://www.drkoop.com*
- Drugstore.com
  Rite-Aid's presence in cyberspace.
     phone: 800-378-4786
     fax: 425-881-9642
     Web: *http://wwwdrugstore.com*
- Emedicine
     Web: *http://www.emedicine.com*
- Federal Telemedicine Gateway
  The U.S. government, especially the military, is doing some of
  the most exciting work in telemedicine today. This portal
  provides one-stop access to everything the government is
  doing.
     Web: *http://www.tmgateway.org*
- *Ferguson Report: The Newsletter of Consumer Health
  Informatics and Online Health*
  Six issues per year.
     3805 Stevenson
     Austin, TX 78703
     phone: 512-474-1141
     fax: 512-474-8444
     subscriptions: 800-219-2057
     Web: *www.doctom@doctom.com*

- Franklin County Health Network
  Web: *http://www.fchn.org*
- Greater Detroit Area Health Council, Inc.
  A community-based healthcare coalition that maintains a consumer-oriented Website rich with local and national resources.
  > 333 W. Fort St.—Suite 1500
  > Detroit, MI 48226-3156
  > phone: 313-963-4990
  > fax: 313-963-4668
  > Web: *www.gdahc.org*
- Harvard Medical Web Home Page
  A good starting point, with links to far-flung medical resources.
  Web: *http://www.med.harvard.edu/*
- Health Gate
  Web: *http://www.healthgate.com*
- Health Information and Application Working Group (HIAWG)
  > Health Level Seven (HL-7)
  > 3300 Washtenaw Ave., Suite 227
  > Ann Arbor, MI 48104
  > phone: 313-677-7777
  > fax: 313-677-6622
  > Web: *www.mcis.duke.edu/ftp/standards.html*
- *Health Management Technology*
  There is a lot about the nuts and bolts of healthcare information technology in this monthly magazine.
  > Nelson Publishing, Inc.
  > 2500 Tamiami Trail North
  > Nokomis, FL 34275
  > phone: 941-966-9521
- Health on the Net
  International foundation dedicated to using the Internet and related technologies to benefit health and medicine. Provides access to Medline, support communities, galleries of images, conferences, and other health information resources.
  Web: *www.hon.ch/home.html*

- *Health Online: How to Find Health Information, Support Groups, and Self-Help Communities in Cyberspace*
    by Tom Ferguson, M.D.
    Reading, Mass.: Addison-Wesley Publishing Company, 1996
- Health Web
  Reliable directory of health information. Links selected by librarians.
    Web: *http://healthweb.org*
- *Healthcare Informatics*
  Monthly magazine on the healthcare informatics industry. Good columnists.
    4530 W. 77th St., Suite 350
    Minneapolis, MN 55435
    phone: 800-525-5003
- Healthcare Informatics Standards Board (HISB)
    Web: *http://web.ansi.org/rooms/room_41/*
- Healthcare Information and Management System Society (HIMSS)
  Famous for its monster annual meeting, swarming with exhibitors and attendees. Pronounced "hymns."
    220 E. Ohio St., Suite 600
    Chicago, IL 60611
    phone: 312-684-4467
    fax: 312-664-6143
    Web: *www.hmss.org*
- Healthfinder
  This site is a service of the U.S. Department of Health and Human Services. It provides links to a wide range of consumer health sites.
    Web: *http://www.healthfinder.gov*
- HealthWorld Online
  Alternative medicine site for consumers.
    Web: *www.healthworld.com*
- HIAWG   See Health Information and Application Working Group.
- HISB   See Healthcare Informatics Standards Board.
- HL-7   See Health Level Seven.
- HIMSS   See Healthcare Information and Management System Society.

- IEEE   See Institute of Electrical and Electronics Engineers.
- *Infocare: Information Strategies for Managed Care*
  Managed care is one place in healthcare where information technology is most mission-critical. This bimonthly magazine reflects that reality.
     4530 W. 77th St., Suite 350
     Minneapolis, MN 55435
     phone: 612-835-3222
     fax: 612-835-3460
     Web: *www.incare.com*
- Institute of Electrical and Electronics Engineers (IEEE)
     445 Hoes Lane, Box 1331
     Piscataway, NJ 08855-1331
     phone: 908-562-3800
     fax: 908-562-1571
     Web: *www.standards.ieee.org*
- Intel Corporation
     Web: *www.intel.com*
- International Organization for Standardization (ISO)
     1, rue de Varembé
     Case postale 56
     CH-1211 Genève 20
     Switzerland
     phone: 41 22 749 01 11
     fax: 41 22 733 34 30
     Web: *www.iso.ch /*
- Internet Dermatology Society
  Dermatology is one of the medical specialties best suited for telemedicine. Learn why and how at this site with extensive, worldwide links.
     Web: *http: / / telemedicine.org*
- Internet Mental Health
  A comprehensive source of information on psychiatric disorders.
     Web: *http: / / www.mentalhealth.com /*
- ISO   See International Organization for Standardization.

- *Journal of the American Medical Informatics Association*
  Bimonthly cutting-edge medical informatics journal.
  > Hanley & Belfus, Inc.
  > 210 S. 13th St.
  > Philadelphia, PA 19107
  > phone: 215-546-7293
- *Journal of Computer Aided Surgery*
  Official journal of the International Society for Computer
  Aided Surgery. As close to science fiction as telemedicine gets.
  > Web: *http://jws-edcc.interscience.wiley.com/cas/*
- Legamed, Inc.
  Annual compendium and quarterly newsletter on the law of
  telemedicine.
  > Legamed, Inc.
  > 8364 Six Forks Road, Suite 104
  > Raleigh, NC 27615
  > phone: 919-676-1137
  > Web: *http://www.legamed.com*
- MDConsult
  Subscribers can search multiple medical texts and journals,
  MEDLINE, and other databases.
  > Web: *www.mdconsult.com*
- Medcast
  This is a Web-based subscription service, primarily for
  physicians, which allows them to customize the medical
  information they want to receive regularly.
  > Web: *http://www.medcast.com/*
- Medscape
  This site offers the Web's largest collection of full-text medical
  articles, conference listings, continuing medical information
  offerings, access to NLM databases, a huge drug-disease
  database, "Journal Scan" summaries of the most recent
  medical literature, and free E-mail, all free of charge to
  physicians.
  > Web: *http://www.medscape.com*
  > E-mail: *blackwell@mail.medscape.com*
- Medsite
  Medical search engine that rates and reviews thousands of
  sites.
  > Web: *www.medsite.com*

- MedWebPlus
  Extensive links to medical information resources worldwide,
  including alternative medicine.
  Web: *http://medwebplus.com*
- Micromedex
  Purveyors of one of the widest arrays of information systems,
  mostly CD-ROM based, focused on the emergency
  department.
  6200 S. Syracuse Way, Suite 300
  Englewood, CO 80111-4740
  phone: 800-525-9083
  fax: 303-486-4740
  Web: *http://www.micromedex.com*
- Microsoft
  One Microsoft Way, Bldg. #8
  North Office 2211
  Redmond, WA 98052
  Web: *www.microsoft.com*
- National Center for Complementary and Alternative
  Medicine
  The National Institutes of Health's foray into alternative
  medicine has concentrated on establishing a scientific basis for
  evaluating nontraditional medicine. This site is their gateway,
  including a huge citation list and bibliography.
  Web: *http://altmed.od.nih.gov/*
- National Computer Security Association
  The name says it all.
  1200 Walnut Bottom Rd.
  Carlisle, PA 17013
  phone: 717-258-1816
  fax: 717-243-8642
  Web: *www.ncsa.com*
- National Council on Quality Assurance (NCQA)
  2000 L St. N.W., Suite 500
  Washington, DC 20036
  phone: 202-955-3500
  fax: 202-955-3599
  Web: *www.ncqa.org*

- National Guideline Clearinghouse (NGC)
  Federally maintained site that contains hundreds of clinical
  practice guidelines gathered from diverse sources.
      phone: 301-594-4042
      Web: *http://www.guideline.gov*
- National Institutes of Health—Consumer Health Information
  A wide range of high-quality information for laypeople.
      Web: *http://www.nih.gov/health/consumer/coincd.htm*
- National Institute for Standards and Technology (NIST)
      100 Bureau Dr.
      Gaithersburg, MD 20899-0001
      phone: 301-975-6478
      Web: *www.nist.gov/*
- National Library of Medicine (NLM)
      8600 Rockville Pike
      Bethesda, MD 20299
      phone: 888-346-3656
      Web: *http://www.nlm.nih.gov/*
  The NLM's free portal to MEDLINE and other medical
  databases:
      Web: *www.index.nlm.nih.gov/databases/freemedl.html*
- National Women's Health Information Center
  A site with extensive information on women's health provided
  for laypeople by the U.S. Public Health Service.
      Web: *http://www.4women.gov*
- NCQA   See National Council on Quality Assurance.
- New York Online Access to Health
  Directory of health sites. A good place to find reliable sources.
      Web: *http://www.noah.cuny.edu*
- Netscape
      Netscape World Headquarters
      501 Middlefield Rd.
      Mountain View, CA 94043
      phone: 650-254-1900
      fax: 650-528-4124
      Web: *http://home.netscape.com*
- NGC   See National Guideline Clearinghouse.
- NIST   See National Institute for Standards and Technology.
- NLM   See National Library of Medicine.

- OnHealth
  A good source for reliable healthcare information for the consumer.
  Web: *www.OnHealth.com*
- PDQ
  The National Cancer Institute's comprehensive database.
  Web: *http://cancerlit.nci.nih.gov/pdq.htm*
- Phase Forward, Inc.
  610 Lincoln St.
  Waltham, MA 02451
  phone: 888-703-1122
  fax: 781-890-4848
  Web: *www.phaseforward.com*
- Physicians' Online Network
  Huge Internet community with open discussions and forums for physicians.
  Web: *www.po.com*
- Planet Rx
  A bellwether site that shows the future of on-line marketing of healthcare items, including information and answers to questions.
  349 Oyster Point Blvd., Suite 201
  South San Francisco, CA 94080
  phone: 650-616-1500
  fax: 650-616-1585
  Web: *www.planetrx.com*
- PubMed
  The National Library of Medicine's site with access to the nine million citations of MEDLINE plus links to on-line journals and other databases.
  Web: *http://www.ncbi.nlm.nih.gov/pubmed/*
- Quackwatch
  Site maintained by a nonprofit corporation whose mission is to combat health fraud and myth.
  Web: *www.quackwatch.com*
- A Starter Set of Internal Medicine Bookmarks
  Compiled by Dr. Jerry Osheroff of the American College of Physicians. A good starting point for finding medical sites on the Web.
  Web: *http://www.acponline.org/computer/ccp/bookmark*

- Sun Microsystems, Inc.
  901 San Antonio Rd.
  Palo Alto, CA 94303
  phone: 800-555-9786
  Web: *http://www.sun.com/*
- TATRC   See Telemedicine and Advanced Technology
  Research Center.
- Tech Encyclopedia
  An on-line glossary of technical terms.
  Web: *http://www.techweb.com/encyclopedia/*
- *Teleconference: The Magazine of Collaborative
  Communications*
  Bimonthly magazine, not just about healthcare. Main focus is
  on hardware.
  210 Sandpointe Ave., Suite 600
  Santa Ana, CA 92707
  phone: 714-513-8400
  fax: 714-513-8632
  Web: *www.teleconferencemagazine.com*
- *Telehealth Magazine: Strategies for Communications &
  Information Management*
  Bimonthly magazine with annual buyer's guide.
  Miller Freeman, Inc.
  600 Harrison St.
  San Francisco, CA 94107
  phone: 415-905-2134
  fax: 415-905-2235
  Web: *http//www.telehealthmag.com*
- Telemedicine and Advanced Technology Research Center
  (TATRC)
  Web: *http://www.tatrc.org/*
- Telemedicine Information Exchange
  Global navigation tool for telemedicine information.
  Web: *http://telemed.org*
- *Telemedicine Journal*
  Official publication of the American Telemedicine Association.
  Mary Ann Liebert, Inc.
  2 Madison Avenue
  Larchmont, NY 10538-1962
  phone: 914-834-3100
  fax: 914-834-3582
  Web: *http://www.liebertpub.com*

- Telemedicine newsgroup
  Join the electronic village.
      E-mail: *news:sci.med.telemedicine*
- Telemedicine and the Law
  Site maintained by the Washington D.C. law firm: Arent, Fox,
  Kintner, Plotkin & Kahn.
      Web: *http://www.arentfox.com/*
- *Telemedicine: Practicing in the Information Age*
  A survey of the field.
      by S.F. Viegas and Kim Dunn, eds.
      New York: Lippincott-Raven, 1998
- *A Telemedicine Primer: Understanding the Issues*
  The basics of developing a telemedicine program.
      by Jim Reid
      Virginia A. Ostendorf, Inc.
      P.O. Box 2896
      Littleton, CO 80161-2896
      phone: 303-797-3131
      fax: 303-797-3524
- Telemedicine Resources
  An extensive set of links maintained by the Image Computing
  Systems Laboratory of the University of Washington.
      Web: *http://icsl.ee.washington.edu/~cabralje/*
      tmresources.html
- *Telemedicine: Theory and Practice*
  A multi-authored survey of the field, written by some of the
  brightest lights in telemedicine.
      by Rashid L. Bashur, Jay H. Sanders, and Gary W.
      Shannon, eds.
      Springfield, Ill.: Charles C. Thomas Publisher, Ltd., 1997
      Web: *http:ccthomas.com*
- *Telemedicine Today: Where Telecommunications and*
  Healthcare Converge
  Bimonthly magazine on telemedicine with annual buyers'
  guide.
      PO Box 11122
      Shawnee Mission, KS 66207-1122
      phone: 913-338-1496
      fax: 913-338-3631
      Web: *www.telemedtoday.com*

- Virtual Hospital Home Page
  Pioneering site from the University of Iowa includes
  multimedia, texts, teaching files, clinical guidelines and
  publications.
     Web: *http://indy.radiology.uiowa.edu/Virtual-
     hospital.html*
- Virtual Lecture Hall
  On-line continuing medical education (CME)
     Web: *http://www.vlh.com*
- Visible Human Project
  The Visible Human Project sliced a male and a female human
  cadaver into sub-millimeter sections and recorded the images
  digitally, allowing any sort of three-dimensional reconstruction
  or "fly-through" that can be imagined. The images generated
  from this database have done more to illustrate the future of
  medical technology than any words could.
     Web: *http://www.nlm.gov/research/visible/
     visible_human.html*
- W3C   See World Wide Web Consortium.
- WebMD
  A comprehensive site with diverse information for consumers
  and health professionals, with many support services under
  development.
     Web: *http://www.webmd.com*
- Wellness Web
  Sensible information for laypeople on traditional medicine,
  alternative medicine, nutrition, exercise, and health
  promotion.
     Web: *http://www.wellweb.com/default.asp*
- Wired
  The hippest print magazine on e-culture. Monthly.
     520 3rd St., 4th Floor
     San Francisco, CA 94107-1815
     phone: 415-276-5000
     E-mail: *editor@wired.com*
     subscriptions: PO Box 55689
     Boulder, CO 80322-5689
     800-SO-WIRED; 303-945-1910; fax: 303-604-7455;
     Web: *wired@neodata.com*

- World Wide Web Consortium (W3C)
    Massachusetts Institute of Technology
    Laboratory for Computer Science
    545 Technology Square
    Cambridge, MA 02139
    phone: 617-253-2613
    fax: 617-258-5999
    Web: *www.w3.org/*
- WWW Virtual Library
  A gateway to medical sites throughout the world.
    Web: *http://www.ohsu.edu/cliniweb/wwwvl/all.html*
- Yahoo HealthMedicine
  Sub-index of medical sites by one of the major Internet
  gateways.
    Web: *http://dir.yahoo.com/Health/Medicine/*

9

Glossary

access network   A connection that allows users of a small remote computer to take advantage of a larger system by tapping into its **backbone.**

ACR-NEMA   See **American College of Radiology and the National Equipment Manufacturers' Association.**

ActiveX   The **Microsoft** Corporation's answer to **Java.**

address   The unique identifier, listed as a combination of letters and numbers, that allows a particular site, machine, or person to be located in an electronic network.

admission-discharge-transfer system (ADT)   Software used by hospitals to keep track of patients throughout their stay.

ADSL   See **asymmetric digital subscriber line.**

ADT   See **admission-discharge-transfer system.**

AI   See **artificial intelligence.**

algorithm   A defined set of rules, usually of a branching structure, that guide a program or a user to a logical endpoint. Branch points or nodes may represent answers to questions or conditions.

alpha site   The location where a product is first tested. With electronics, alpha sites are usually closely related to where the product has been developed. Few others would put up with the hassles of getting an untested system up and running. See **beta site.**

American College of Radiology and the National Equipment Manufacturers' Association (ACR-NEMA) The source of jointly-developed standards for digital radiography equipment.

American National Standards Institute (ANSI) The U.S. member of the **International Standards Organization** that works to establish electronic data standards.

American Standard Code for Information Interchange (ASCII) The standard coding scheme that assigns numeric values to letters, numbers, punctuation marks, and control characters. ASCII values are each seven-bit codes, with an eighth parity bit used for error checking.

analog In contrast to **digital** signals, which are encoded strings of discrete values, analog signals vary continuously. A turntable, for example, puts out an analog signal, generated by the hills and valleys continuously traversed by its needle in the record groove.

ANSI See **American National Standards Institute.**

Apple Cupertino, California based firm which, with its Macintosh machines, pioneered in commercialization of concepts of user friendliness in personal computers, including the virtual **desktop, what you see is what you get (WYSIWYG), and the graphical user interface (GUI).** Through marketing missteps and aggressive competition by arch-rival Microsoft's Windows system, Apple's share of the PC market plummeted, holding onto niches in publishing and education. The firm showed renewed vigor in 1998, with the return of its founding CEO, Steven Jobs.

applet A small program out of which larger programs can be constructed. Applets may be transmitted on networks and loaded onto receiving machines with programs to be executed. **ActiveX** and **Java** are applet-based languages.

application Software designed to perform a specific function, as opposed to system software, which runs the machines themselves. Application software may do word processing, graphics, music, or a nearly limitless host of other functions.

application server A **file server** optimized for a specific task such as management of a particular database or communications network.

architecture When referring to hardware, the architecture is the actual structure of a system, identifying which machines are connected to each other via what kinds of connections. With software, architecture refers to the overall logical plan.

archiving Saving data for later reference. Archived data may not be as immediately accessible as current data.

artificial intelligence The science of getting electronic machines to "reason" by making deductions, recognizing patterns, or other modes of replicating human uses of data.

ASCII See **American Standard Code for Information Interchange.**

Association of Telemedicine Service Providers (ATSP) The premier industry group for telemedicine, founded in 1997.

asymmetric digital subscriber line (ADSL) A way of using digital signals to provide higher bandwidth on a **twisted pair** of copper wires. Can currently transmit data at up to 6 Mbps.

asynchronous transfer mode (ATM) A digital network standard that provides high bandwidth for transmitting multiple types of data. Messages are broken down and sent in **packets** which traverse the network independently, to be reconstructed in the proper sequence at the receiving station.

ATM See **asynchronous transfer mode.**

ATSP See **Association of Telemedicine Service Providers.**

audit trail An electronic record showing access and changes to data in a system. In accounting, this may allow detailed tracing and reconstruction of transactions. It can also function as a security feature that provides a log detailing which users accessed which files at what times.

authentication One of the processes involved in security. A set of software protocols assuring that sources of electronic messages are who they say they are and verifying the integrity of the message.

backbone The main, high-speed electronic conduit that carries the highest volume of electronic messages in a system. Today, most commonly fiberoptic cable.

back-up The process of duplicating data or programs on a second storage device as insurance against losing them in a system failure.

bandwidth A measure of the raw carrying capacity of an electronic channel. The higher the bandwidth, the more data can be transmitted in the same amount of time. Today bandwidth is often the critical factor in limiting the performance of networked systems. Measured in **bps, bits per second.**

baseband transmission A single channel transmission system used mostly in **local area networks,** including **Ethernet.**

BBS See **bulletin board system.**

benchmarking Testing of the actual performance of a system in comparison to relevant norms and standards.

beta site After most of the **bugs** are worked out at an **alpha site,** systems are installed for real-world testing at beta sites. Depending on the system and its builders, beta testing can be an opportunity to get an early crack at a good product under favorable terms or a horror of compounding errors.

bigger or faster is better (BOFIB) Self-explanatory phrase in electronics circles.

biosensors Electronic devices that convert biologic inputs, such as blood pressure, joint position, or brain waves, into electronic outputs.

bit The smallest unit of information. Contraction of "binary digit"—a 1 or a 0, represented by "on" or "off" of a digital switch.

bit depth   A term used in digital imaging. Each point in the image is specified by a set of numbers that locate it in space. The number of bits available to describe some characteristic of that point, such as color, is referred to as the bit depth.

bits per second (bps)   Unit for measuring the speed of data transmission. See also **Kbps** and **Mbps.**

BOFIB   See **bigger or faster is better.**

bookmark   An electronic signpost feature of most web browsers, which allows users to save Internet addresses so they can return to the sites easily.

Boolean   A type of algebra, developed in the nineteenth century by George Boole, a British mathematician. It represents logical propositions with abstract symbols. AND, OR, and NOT are three of the Boolean operators which lie at the foundation of software construction.

boot   The steps that a computer goes through when it starts up, including loading parts of the **operating system** into **RAM,** checking what **peripheral devices** are connected, testing circuits, etc.

bot   See **intelligent agent.**

bridge   An electronic switch that allows users from multiple sites to participate in an audio or video conference.

broadband communications   Communication requiring high bandwidth for accomplishment, such as real-time, full motion video.

broadband network   Capable of transmission rates of at least 1.5 **Mbps.**

browser   A program that contains the communication software which allows the user to explore a network that uses Internet protocols, including the Internet itself. Browsers may have multiple additional features such as electronic mail, **newsgroup** access, etc. Netscape Navigator and Internet Explorer are the two most popular browsers.

bug   A glitch, usually referring to software. The term was coined by Thomas Edison in 1878 to describe little flaws that needed to be worked out of an invention or process. Others attribute the modern use of this term to the 1940s when a grasshopper (in some versions, a moth) was found to have shorted out a relay in ENIAC, the progenitor of all electronic computers.

bulletin board system (BBS)   A sort of electronic meeting place where messages can be placed and retrieved. BBSs may become hosts for ongoing discussions, usually based upon a common interest of the participants. There are thousands of them on the Internet.

bus   A central, high transmission capacity pathway within an information processing device or a network.

bus topology   A network architecture in which connections to machines branch off of a main, linear, high-bandwidth conduit.

byte   The next bigger measure of information content than a **bit.** A byte is eight binary digits, capable of expressing 256 (2^8) different values or corresponding states.

C/C++ Common programming languages. C was first designed to implement the **Unix** operating system. It is one of the most commonly used programming languages for commercial software. C++ is a direct descendant, designed for use with **object-oriented technology. Java** can also trace its lineage to C.

call-back A security technique for systems accessed by modems. A prospective client dials in to the system, which hangs up, compares the client to a list of authorized users and, if the client passes muster, calls back and allows a log-in (with password, of course).

CBT See **computer-based training.**

CCD See **charge coupled device.**

CD-ROM See **compact disk, read-only memory.**

cell switch A device that transmits data cells, packets of information of fixed size, in a continuous stream over a fixed path. Compare to **frame relay.**

centralized computing Traditional data management architecture where a mainframe or mid-range computer does most of an organization's information processing. Compare to **distributed computing.**

central processing unit (CPU) The "guts" of a computer. This chip or group of chips does the actual calculating.

certification authority Part of a security system which controls access to an information network by managing users' access privileges and verifying their identity at log-in.

chaos theory A branch of mathematics and statistical mechanics that describes the behavior of complex systems. It distinguishes orderly systems, such as bouncing billiard balls, from chaotic systems, such as the weather, and describes how to discern the possibility of patterns in the latter. Computer simulations are essential tools for exploring models of chaotic systems.

charge coupled device (CCD) A specialized silicon chip which turns light into digital electrical signals. Among their uses, CCDs are the receivers behind the lens of video cameras.

chat group A group that carries on a discussion in **cyberspace.**

CHIN See **community health information network.**

chip A wafer, usually of silicon, upon which are embossed the circuits that are the basis of the electronics industry. The technology and materials of production change at a rapid rate. See **Moore's Law.**

client A computer for use by end-users that sends and receives data through a **server.** A **thin client** is a computer with limited capabilities for independent processing. A fat client brings more of the computing power and program to the interchange with a server. When a Web **browser** requests data from a server, its host computer becomes a client of that machine.

client/server The network architecture that specifies some computers for processing by end-users **(clients)** and some for holding data and providing networking functions **(servers).** The Internet employs a client/server approach.

CLIMS   See **clinical laboratory information management system.**

clinical decision support   The capability of a system to provide data to clinicians based on rule-based triggers. Examples include: automatic notification of "panic" laboratory values or of drug interactions and tailored prompts for patient monitoring based on new orders.

clinical laboratory information management system   An electronic system that collects, organizes, reports, and stores patient laboratory data.

clock speed   Electronic computers break complex problems down into tiny steps in order to solve them. Because electrons move at the speed of light, they can take each step in a tiny amount of time. A clock, which serves as the pacemaker at the heart of a **CPU,** determines the speed at which each calculation cycle occurs. The faster the clock speed, the faster and more powerful the computer.

clone   A computing device produced and sold, usually at a discount, that functions essentially identical to the device of an original manufacturer.

COTS   Commercial off-the-shelf.

coaxial cable   The electronic cable that cable television companies use to bring signals to subscribers and that forms the backbone for some computer networks, including Ethernet. Called "coaxial" because it consists of an inner wire and an outer conducting sheath, both sharing the same axis. Capable of carrying up to 140 Mbps. Slang term, "coax," pronounced "co-ax."

code   Refers to software instructions in programming language. May also refer to the output of an **encryption** process.

codec   See **coder/decoder.**

coder/decoder (codec)   On the sending side, this device converts video data into a digital signal for transmission. On the receiving side it turns the signal back into a video signal. **Compression** algorithms reduce the bandwidth necessary to transmit the signal. See **modem.**

common object request broker architecture (CORBA)   A standard for **object-oriented technology** programming which allows data to be shared among applications.

community health information network (CHIN)   An organization providing connections that allow providers, payors, and purchasers to exchange electronically financial and clinical healthcare information within a geographic region.

compact disk, read-only memory (CD-ROM)   The familiar silvery disks used to record and play back music. Called "read-only" because, once recorded, the information it contains is not erasable or changeable. Also used to record data. One disk holds about 660 MB.

compiler   Computer software which translates **programming languages,** used by people, into **machine language,** used directly by a computer.

compression   The process of compacting data to be transmitted over a channel of limited **bandwidth.** For example, compression routines that eliminate the need to transmit unchanging picture background can reduce the bandwidth needed to transmit full motion video up to 200 times.

computed radiography A medical imaging system that has been digitized, from data acquisition to storage to transmission to access to analysis.

computer-based patient record (CPR) See **electronic medical record (EMR).**

The Computer-based Patient Record Institute (CPRI) Forum for the healthcare community to promote the **CPR.**

computer-based training (CBT) Automated training that takes advantage of computers' ability to support interactive multimedia techniques. In certain realms, well-designed CBT may eliminate or greatly reduce the need for human teachers.

computerized medical record See **electronic medical record.**

consumer health informatics Term coined by Tom Ferguson, M.D. (see pages 76 and 77) to describe how laypeople inform themselves about health and medicine: what resources they use and how they use them (e.g., print and electronic information and support groups, including those that are based electronically).

convergence The concept that computers and electronic communications media are coevolving into common multipurpose devices. Combination printer/copier/phone/fax machines and pager/phone/personal digital assistants are two current examples of this phenomenon, which is expected to accelerate under pressure of competition to meet consumer needs. Likewise, mostly due to mergers and buyouts, the companies that provide electronic devices and communication services are converging into huge, multifaceted organizations that furnish and move data via multiple technologies.

cookie Data inserted by a **server** into a **browser** which then resides temporarily in the browser, storing information like **passwords,** preferences, and **bookmarks.** Until the cookie expires, its information will be available to smooth the interaction whenever the browser re-accesses that server.

CORBA See **common object request broker architecture.**

cost-benefit Ratio of the cost of acquiring a new machine or method to the economic benefit it is likely to produce over time.

cost-effectiveness This economic concept allows comparison of the different costs of producing a desired outcome with different inputs.

COTS See **commercial off-the-shelf.**

CPR See **computer-based patient record.**

CPRI See **The Computer-based Patient Record Institute.**

CPU See **central processing unit.**

CR See **computed radiography.**

crash When an electronic device or system stops working, sometimes catastrophically, it is said to crash. The term originates from failing hard drives, where the read/write head can actually crash into the disk, destroying its data.

cryptography   The science of codes and ciphers.

cybernetics   A field developed in the 1950s by Norbert Weiner, an MIT mathematician. Its goal is to understand how to use information to control systems, ranging from thermostats to robots. Feedback is a cybernetic concept.

cyberspace   Term coined by William Gibson in his 1984 science fiction novel *Neuromancer* to describe the virtual world spawned by networked complex electronic systems. Cyberspace is to networked computers what innerspace is to human brains.

cycle time   How long it takes for a new product to come to market and displace the previous one. Cycle times are getting shorter, especially in the electronics industry. See **Moore's Law.**

data   The raw material that computing machines collect, massage, manipulate, store, and report. Regardless of the form in which they enter, data must be converted to a digital form, numbers, before they can be handled by a digital computer. Singular, datum.

database   Both the software structure used to keep data in an orderly, usable format and the data themselves, once they have been entered into the file.

data dictionary   The precise description of each data element. Development of a data dictionary is the first step in constructing a **database.**

data element   A specific piece of information or required content, such as patient name or blood glucose level.

data entry   Getting information into the system, whether by **keyboard, OCR, biosensor, speech recognition, CCD,** or any other means. Often the slow step in automating a process.

data mart   A database organized for easy searching. It is a step more structured than a **data warehouse,** upon which the mart may reside.

data mining   The process of extracting information from data. The software equivalent of asking and answering questions. Also called **drilling down** on the data.

data repository   The least structured form of a database. The structure into which raw data are dumped from multiple sources.

data warehouse   Intermediate in structure between a **data repository** and **data mart,** where data have been aggregated enough for **mining** but not refined to the extent as in a data mart.

debugging   The process of finding and repairing errors in software code. See **bug.**

decision support   The use of information, derived from system data, to help make strategic decisions.

default   In a **data dictionary,** what is filled in if a data item is left blank. For example, if the date field is not completed as a record is entered, the system may be set to default to the current date.

desktop The way of representing computer files in most **GUI** systems, in which the computer display is organized as a personal work space containing, for example, a filing cabinet, writing tools, and accounting tools. Also, the standard size, nonportable personal computer is a desktop model.

developer Usually refers to an individual who writes software that translates users' needs into a code understood by a machine.

dial-up Telecommunication based on **POTS,** with connections made by using regular phone numbers.

DICOM See **digital image and communications in medicine.**

digital The dominant branch of electronic computing based upon discrete numbers usually represented as strings of zeroes and ones, equivalent to switches being turned off or on. Compare to **analog,** where numbers are represented by continuous, nondiscrete quantities.

digital certificate A subset of encryption technology that allows receivers to confirm the authenticity of an electronic message.

digital dictation A system that stores voice files digitally, which allows more flexible archiving and access. Another advantage of digitized files is that they allow transcriptionists to slow down or speed up the replay rate without distorting the sound of the voice as with analog systems.

digital image and communications in medicine (DICOM) The collection of industry standards for communication between medical imaging devices.

digital signature A security technique that allows, by appropriate use of password or encryption, for an individual to give a verifiable imprimatur to a document without physically having to append a handwritten signature.

digital subscriber line (DSL) A type of phone connection which is five times faster than **ISDN.** DSL allows simultaneous digital and voice transmission on the same line.

digital versatile disk (DVD) An optical disk format which stores up to fourteen times more information than a **CD-ROM.** It can be used for data, audio, or video. One DVD can store a full-length film. This technology could soon be exploited to hold up to 17 **GB** per disk.

disease management An approach, developed under the stimulus of capitated insurance plans, to improve the care of complex, chronic diseases such as diabetes or asthma across the continuum of care—from self-care at home to discharge planning immediately after hospitalization. Good, accessible data are especially critical to disease management.

disintermediation A process, greatly facilitated by electronic communication, whereby providers and consumers of goods or services are directly in contact, leaving out the middlemen and, theoretically, making the market more efficient.

diskless workstation A **thin client** computer which downloads the programs it requires from a server as it needs them and discards them when finished.

disk operating system (DOS)   The core system software for any personal computer. **Microsoft**'s version, MS-DOS, became a dominant force when IBM selected it as the operating system for their personal computers in 1980. Thereafter the fame and fortune of Bill Gates, Microsoft's founder, was guaranteed. MS-DOS has been supplanted by the more user-friendly **Windows.** Its main competitor is **Apple's Macintosh** operating system.

distributed computing   Network architecture which spreads computing power and duties out among machines, rather than having the power primarily reside in a big server or mainframe computer. Distributed computing is a cheap way to add power and flexibility to a system but presents challenges in terms of complexity, maintenance, and coordination. Compare to **centralized computing.**

DNS   See **domain name service.**

document imaging   Conversion of paper documents to scanned images for storage in a computer system. See **scanning.**

domain   A set of network addresses, such as ".can" for Canada and ".edu" for education institutions. The next lower domain refers to a particular company or institution, and so on until a particular addressee is specified. For example, *www.healthedgroup.com* is the McGraw-Hill webpage that leads to a listing of this book.

domain name service (DNS)   The rules whereby the Internet is divided into hierarchical domains. Stakes can be high in the domain name system. For example, Tuvalu, a tiny island in the South Pacific, stands to make millions by licensing use of its domain, ".tv" to Internet sites that have something to do with television.

DOS   See **disk operating system.**

download   The process of bringing information or programs into a computing device. The opposite of **upload.**

DSL   See **digital subscriber line.**

drilling down   See **data mining.**

dumb terminal   The lowliest of computers tied into a network. Basically, a keyboard and a monitor screen lacking internal memory. Dumb terminals use computing resources that reside elsewhere in the network.

duplex audio   The ability of participants at both ends of a conference to speak simultaneously, as in a phone call. If the connection will only allow one party to speak at a time, this is half-duplex.

duplexing   Sending two electronic signals simultaneously over the same line. It essentially doubles the amount of information that can be transmitted per unit of time. Also a synonym for **mirroring.**

DVD   See **digital versatile disk.**

e-commerce   Business conducted via electronic communications.

EDI   See **electronic data interchange.**

electronic data interchange (EDI) Electronic transmission of data between computers.

electronic mail (E-mail) A set of protocols that allows users to exchange electronic messages which they can pick up at will. E-mail is the archetypal **store-and-forward** application.

electronic medical record (EMR) The ideal is an all-electronic (i.e., paperless) archive of a patient's medical data—accessible, with authorization, from anywhere. The record itself does not have to reside on one machine. It may be an organized look at data about one patient collected from multiple sources, all pulled together under a **universal patient identifier.**

E-mail See **electronic mail.**

EMR See **electronic medical record.**

encryption A set of techniques that allows confidentiality to be preserved, identities to be confirmed, documents to be authenticated, and a host of other security functions to be performed.

enterprisewide network A network that connects together every computer in an organization. A mission critical piece to the information systems strategy of integrated care delivery systems.

environment In the computer world, the environment is the totality of hardware, software, connections, and protocols in which the system functions.

Ethernet A commonly employed networking system designed by the Xerox Corporation that allows computers that are wired together to exchange data. Capable of 10 to 100 **Mbps** transmission.

executable Means that a piece of software can be run on a certain **platform.**

executive information system Software that allows an administrator to draw together data from various sources in an organization to assist in decision making.

expert system A software routine which is capable of assisting decision making, much as a human expert would. A branch of **artificial intelligence.**

eXtensible Markup Language (XML) The likely successor to **HTML** being developed by the **W3C.** A step-up in power, versatility, and ease of use.

extranet Use of the Internet to provide communication services for an organization. Security issues in this public medium can be addressed by **encryption,** rather than by owning secure private lines. See **intranet.**

FDDI See **fiber distributed data interface.**

fiber distributed data interface (FDDI) A fiberoptic network specification that currently allows for transmission rates of up to 100 **Mbps.**

fiberoptic Glass fibers that conduct light for data transmission, which provides a much broader **bandwidth** than **twisted pair** or **coaxial cable.** Because this technology requires converting electrical signals to light impulses and back, it is significantly more challenging than purely electrical systems but in many situations well worth the effort for the increment in bandwidth. Today, fiberoptics form the **backbone** of most large networks.

file   A group of data that belong together, such as the file that is the medical record of an individual or the file that is the list of all patients of a particular clinic. A file may contain data and/or programs and/or other files.

file server   A network computer that stores data and makes it accessible to other computers **(clients).**

file transfer protocol (FTP)   Electronic rules, part of the overall Internet protocols that allow data to be exchanged between computers.

firewall   A software structure, sometimes also a separate computer, which isolates devices within a network from computers on the outside. The firewall is designed to admit only safe communications from authorized users and keep out intruders.

firmware   Midway between hardware and software. The programs embedded in chips that are not modifiable. Videogame cassettes, which contain all the information necessary to make the game appear on the television screen, are an example of firmware.

flame   To disparage in an electronic message. When flaming becomes two-sided, it can erupt into a flame war. To breach **netiquette** is to invite flaming.

flash memory   Digital chips that retain data after the power is turned off. Used in medical imaging devices and digital cameras. Today's flash memory cards have capacities up to 48 **MB.**

floppy disk   A vinyl disk impregnated with an electronic substrate upon which data can be written and from which they can be read. Carrying around a floppy has become less important as they have fallen out of favor over the last few years. Computers' hard drives have become capable of storing more data and networks now carry data from one machine to another. The most common floppies store about 1.2 **MB.**

formatting   Refers to how data are arranged on a storage disk and how they are displayed or printed by a computer.

frame   Transmission unit for **frame relay.** Also, one still image in a motion picture.

frame rate   The number of frames displayed per second in a video. Standard broadcast television is at 30 frames per second (fps) in the United States and Canada.

frame relay   A method of transmitting data across a digital network in high speed bursts in units called frames. Though it supports data transmission in the range of 56 Kbps to 1.54 Mbps, it is not well suited to audio and video messages in real time because of the discontinuity of data arrival.

FTP   See **file transfer protocol.**

full-motion video   The gold standard in video quality. This requires a rate of 25 to 30 frames per second in order to fool the human eye into seeing continuous motion.

function point analysis A way of quantifying the likely size and cost of developing new software, based upon the broadest outline of its intended function.

fuzzy logic An **artificial intelligence** technique which attempts to mimic human thought by functioning with inexact operations rather than the more precise either/or type categories of standard logic.

gateway This is a starting point onto the World Wide Web. Popular gateways include Yahoo, Excite, Lycos, AltaVista, and InfoSeek. They are loaded with the electronic version of advertising banners, making them valuable properties for the same reason as billboards at the entrances to busy freeways are. Also, the gateway provided by a proxy server is the connection between an internal network and an external one. See **search engine.**

GB See **gigabyte.**

GIF See **graphics interface format.**

gigabyte 1,000,000,000 bytes. A thousand **megabytes.** Commonly abbreviated as GB, such as an 8.0 GB hard drive

Golbus' First Law "No major computer system is ever installed on time, within budget, with the same staff that started it, nor does the project fully do what it's supposed to do."

Gopher A system, developed at the University of Minnesota, that allows one computer to search another computer's files over the Internet. By employing Gopher, a user can review a menu of an archive's holdings then use FTP to download the appropriate files. Graphical Web protocols have greatly eclipsed text-based Gopher as a tool for searching out data.

graphical user interface (GUI) An approach to software invented by Xerox but commercially developed by **Apple** for the **Macintosh** and copied by **Microsoft** for **Windows.** A GUI (pronounced "gooey") gives the computer user a visual representation on the computer screen that can be used to tell the computer what to do. It takes the place of commands, which may be non-intuitive complicated series of keystrokes. GUI has helped make computers dramatically more "user-friendly."

graphics interchange format (GIF) Along with **JPEG,** one of the two most common formats for displaying images on the Web.

Grateful Med The **National Library of Medicine**'s user-friendly software for doing searches of its databases.

GUI See **graphical user interface.**

H.323 The current critical set of standards underpinning multimedia communications.

hacker Hackers use their computers to enter other computer systems where they are not wanted. They may simply come and go just to show they can beat the **firewalls, encryption,** and other roadblocks thrown in their way, or they can do real mischief by corrupting data or even crashing the whole system.

haptic feedback A cornerstone of **virtual reality.** It provides touch and movement sensation back to the operator. This could be engine thrust impulse fed back to a simulator pilot, tissue resistance to a surgeon operating remotely, or joint position to the user of an artificial limb.

hard drive A method of data storage. Data and programs are electronically written onto and read off of a rapidly spinning disk. Most computers have hard drives. Along with internal fans, they cause the whirring you hear when you turn on a personal computer.

hardware Contrasts with **software;** the instructions which run the hardware, the physical electronic devices.

HDTV See **high density television.**

Healthcare Informatics Standards Board (HISB) A group within **ANSI** that works on standards for computer-based patient records.

Health Information and Application Working Group (HIAWG) The part of the U.S. Information Infrastructure Task Force that recommends how the national information infrastructure could be used to benefit healthcare.

Health Level-7 (HL-7) A group establishing standards for electronic interchange of text messages in healthcare such as scheduling, admissions, and discharges.

Health Plan Employer Data and Information Set (HEDIS) A core set of performance measures designed by **NCQA** to assist purchasers of healthcare in assessing and comparing the quality of health plans. Pronounced "heedis."

HEDI See **Health Plan Employer Data and Information Set.**

help desk A critical component of many organizations' information services. The help desk is where users turn—in person, by phone, or by E-mail—to help them make their piece of the system work.

Hertz A measure of frequency in cycles per second. Usually refers to the clock speed of a computer or to the frequency of the wave that carries an electronic signal. See **megahertz.**

HIAWG See **Health Information and Application Working Group.**

high density television (HDTV) High resolution broadcast video, with about four times the vertical resolution of the current standard.

HISB See **Healthcare Informatics Standards Board.**

HL-7 See **Health Level-7.**

home page The starting point for a presence on the Internet. It is the first view seen by somebody who has directed a computer to the main address. A health system's home page, for example, might have the organization's logo on the background with buttons that lead to its individual hospitals, a medical staff directory, a mission statement, a list of services, etc. The home page actually resides as a data file on a server.

hot-link   A "button," usually in the shape of a highlighted word or picture that leads from one Internet site to another. For example, a medical practice might, in the paragraph that describes its hospital affiliations, have hot-links that lead to the home pages of those hospitals. See **hypertext link.**

HTML   See **hypertext markup language.**

http   See **hypertext transfer protocol.**

hub   The machine through which all messages pass, as in a hub-and-spoke **network architecture.** Usually the most powerful computer of the group.

hub-and-spoke   See **star topology.**

hypertext   A way of organizing a document on the computer which links pieces to each other in a sort of three-dimensional topology. Rather than the linear presentation of a conventional text, a hypertext document allows the user to explore it in a fashion that leads from piece to piece via links which connect them to each other in complex ways.

hypertext link   The pointers within a hypertext document which attach pieces to each other, often in a nonlinear way. Hypertext links allow users to follow multiple, individual paths through the material. See **hot-link.**

hypertext markup language (HTML)   The lingua franca of the Internet. A set of electronic protocols that allows different machines, running different operating systems, to exchange and display information intelligibly. See **eXtensible Markup Language.**

hypertext transfer protocol (HTTP)   The electronic routines that allow computers to send and receive hypertext-based documents. See **hypertext markup language.**

ICD-10   See **International Classification of Diseases, 10th Revision.**

icon   A small picture on a computer screen that represents a program, file, or function. Icons are key components of **GUI**s.

IEEE   See **Institute of Electrical and Electronics Engineers.**

IETF   See **Internet Engineering Task Force.**

image   An electronic representation that translates into a sensory picture. Not limited to visual images, though this is the usual reference.

informatics   The applied science of collecting, storing, and retrieving data to support informed decision making.

information   Raw data which has been processed to the point of making some sense.

information appliance   A hardware/software combination that allows a user to access specific information sources, such as the terminals in a library that access only an "electronic card catalog." A low-cost alternative to a fully-outfitted computer.

information resource dictionary system An enterprise-wide software tool that coordinates all of its **data dictionaries** in order to maintain consistent meanings for data throughout the organization.

information superhighway See **National Information Infrastructure.**

information system The combination of hardware, software, people, and data which serve the information needs of an organization.

information theory Developed in the 1940s by Claude Shannon, an electrical engineer at Bell Laboratories. An abstract mathematical view of communications most useful for calculating the performance of electronic devices. Information is rigorously defined as the opposite of randomness and entropy, thereby relating the laws of information theory to the laws of thermodynamics.

infrared (Ir) A part of the spectrum with wavelengths just longer than the red end of visible light. Most useful today for providing wireless links between such devices as entertainment center remote controls and televisions or personal digital assistants and personal computers.

Institute of Electrical and Electronics Engineers (IEEE) The IEEE is the world's largest technical professional society. It has developed and continues to develop many of the accepted standards for electronic products.

integrated services digital network (ISDN) A digital communication protocol that currently allows data to be transmitted at up to 128 Kbps on a single wire.

integration The task of ensuring that all devices in an information system work together and that the data they share is "understood" by all.

Intel Corporation Largest manufacturer of computer chips in the world, including most of the chips that run the Windows operating systems. Intel's market clout is so great that, along with Microsoft's **Windows,** it is considered half of Wintel, the nickname for the consortium that is said to control the world of computing.

intelligent agent An **applet** designed to move from machine to machine seeking out information and making transactions in accord with the needs of the customer. For example, an intelligent agent might be charged to search Internet databases of a number of blood banks, seeking to locate the four units of a certain rare type that are nearest geographically, arrange for their transport, and handle the paperwork and financial transactions. Also called a **bot,** to show analogy to its physical counterpart, the robot.

intelligent optical character reader Software which turns scanned images of characters (letters, numbers, etc.) into digital representations, providing all the benefits of digital data, including categorization, searchability, and reformatting.

interactive voice response Automated audio systems, usually telephone based, which allow the system to fulfill users' needs based upon their responses. Upon returning from the beach, a person could, for example, phone in and direct an education system to play the segment about sunburn by making the correct responses to system queries.

interface Where one system—hardware, software, and/or use—meets another. Interface problems, getting disparate systems to work together, present some of the biggest challenges to **system analysts.**

interface engine A software application which makes development and management of interfaces more manageable.

International Classification of Diseases 10th Revision A World Health Organization enumeration of diseases, injuries, and causes of death. Used in many health data systems to standardize reports and comparisons.

International Standards Organization (ISO) Establishes and coordinates worldwide standards for electronic information exchange.

Internet The overall worldwide network of networks, hardware and software, loosely connected together using standard communications protocols. The precursor to the Internet was ARPANET, funded by the U.S. Department of Defense in 1969 to link four distant computers together as a network. More than anything else, standard communications protocols (electronic rules) are what define the Internet. They are subject to revision by the **IETF,** the international governing body for the Internet.

Internet 2 The next generation Internet, more secure and with higher bandwidth, is still on the drawing boards.

Internet Engineering Task Force (IETF) This is as close as the anarchically-inclined Internet gets to a governing body. A loosely-defined working group which sets standards for Internet protocols.

Internet protocol suite (IPS) The software necessary to connect to the Internet, specifically **TCP/IP** and **FTP.**

Internet service provider (ISP) The entity which connects customers to the Internet via their server. There are thousands of ISPs.

interoperability The ability of two different hardware systems to run the same software, which exponentially reduces system **integration** headaches.

interventional informatics Using information systems to improve patient care in real time. An interventional informatics strategy might be to cue the information system to automatically provide critical information about the patient or disease, or to check certain laboratory parameters at the time of service before executing a prescription order.

intranet When **client/server** architecture and **TCP/IP** are used on an internal network, this network qualifies as an intranet. See **enterprisewide network.**

IP address The four-part number with no more than three digits per part that uniquely identifies every computer on the Internet.

IPS See **internet protocol suite.**

Ir See **infrared.**

ISDN   See **integrated services digital network.**

ISO   See **International Standards Organization .**

ISP   See **Internet service provider.**

IVR   See **interactive voice response.**

Java   An **object-oriented technology** programming language developed by **Sun Microsystems** which has special utility for distributed, Internet-based applications. Composed of **applets** which can be exchanged between computers.

Joint Photographic Expert's Group (JPEG)   This standard, designed by the **ISO,** is one of the two main algorithms used for compressing still images.

JPEG   See **Joint Photographic Expert's Group.**

jukebox   A machine capable of storing massive amounts of data on multiple hard disks. In medical settings it is most commonly used to maintain the enormous databases encoded by electronic imaging systems.

KB   See **kilobyte.**

Kbps   Transmission rate of 1,000 **bits** per second.

key   In **cryptography,** the information which allows a receiver to decode an encrypted message.

keyboard   An input device that translates finger pressure on an array of numbered/lettered buttons into an electronic signal. Today's kids learn keyboarding rather than typing in school.

kilobyte (KB)   1,024 **bytes.**

knowledge base   A way of representing data so that individual concepts are related to each other logically. Sort of a database packed with **artificial intelligence.**

LAN   See **local area network.**

laptop   A portable computer with a full-size or near full-size keyboard and screen. Though they fit in a briefcase, higher-end laptops may do most of the same tasks with the same efficiency as a **desktop** model.

last mile problem   Virtually every home and workplace in America can be connected to the Internet via its telephone wires. Unfortunately, these **twisted pairs** are low **bandwidth.** So, no matter how high speed the **backbone** of the system may be, today the grand majority of users cannot take advantage of it due to the slowness of their personal connection (the last mile). **ISDN, ATM,** microwave and satellite links, and television cable are a few of the competing solutions.

LATA See **local access and transport area.**

learning curve This construct plots effort and payoff over time for an individual or an organization coming to understand and use a new system, machine, or technique. Typically, the effort curve is steep and the payoff curve is shallow at the beginning, meaning a lot of work for little benefit. Hopefully, these parameters reverse later in the course after adoption to provide a payoff.

leased line A phone connection that, for a fee to the **telco,** is dedicated exclusively to traffic of the purchaser.

LEC See **local exchange company.**

legacy system An older electronic system. Such systems usually have the dual problem of being outdated and entrenched. Dealing with legacy systems is one of the biggest headaches for information services managers.

Linux An up-and-coming **operating system,** developed by Linus Torvalds. An **open system** known for its **robustness,** used mainly for **servers,** it has a growing following and commercial importance.

listserv A program that distributes messages to a mailing list on the Internet. Subscribers to a listserv do so to keep up on a field of particular interest. It is one way to tailor the information that one receives to meet one's personal needs. Listserv is a **push** technology. There are tens of thousands of listservs.

local access and transport area (LATA) The region within which a Regional Bell Operating Company or a local exchange company provide telephony services.

local area network (LAN) When computers and other devices at one site are connected together, the result is a LAN. Contrast to **WAN.**

local exchange company (LEC) The local telephone service that connects customers within its service area to each other and to long distance services.

lossless A signal compression method that loses no data. When the signal is reconstructed by the receiver it should be identical with the signal that was sent. Lossless compression requires more bandwidth than **lossy.**

lossy A signal compression algorithm that sacrifices 100% fidelity for the ability to greatly reduce bandwidth. Compare to **lossless.**

Luddite A pejorative term in high-tech circles. It means being against new technology on general principles and carries connotations of being rigid and old-fashioned. The original Luddites got their name from Ned Ludd, leader of a radical group of British weavers who, at the beginning of the Industrial Revolution, correctly perceived the threat of automated looms to their skilled trade. They protested by smashing the new machines. Of course, the Luddites lost their battle against the tidal wave of the Industrial Revolution in short order.

machine language The binary instructions that actually tell a digital machine what to do. Compare to **programming language.**

Macintosh   Apple's **GUI** operating system for personal computers.

mainframe   A big fast computer. Mainframe machines are where electronic computing started, giving way in the 1980s to smaller machines when the economics of microelectronics shifted the focus to powerful personal computers. No matter how well designed and connected their network of personal computers, most large organizations still need the raw computing power of mainframes to do some of their centralized data processing tasks. See centralized computing.

maintenance   The ongoing job of keeping a system running. May be even more complex than installation.

MAN   See metropolitan area network.

master patient index (MPI)   This is critical to any healthcare billing system and the fulcrum of the electronic patient record. An MPI allows every patient datum to be tied to the correct person, stored, and retrieved. **Resolvers**—sophisticated programs which remove data ambiguity, such as multiple name spellings, and assign a unique identifier to each patient—have greatly simplified the job of maintaining an MPI.

MB   See **megabyte.**

Mbps   Transmission rate of 1,000,000 bits per second.

medical information bus (MIB)   The **IEEE** protocol specifies standards for connecting patient monitoring systems with information systems.

medium   This refers to the communication substrate upon which information is projected. There are hard copy media—such as magazines, newspapers, paintings, and conventional X rays—and electronic media—such as radio, television, CD, Internet, and digital radiology. Media should be used so as to exploit their strengths while taking into account their limitations. For example, in the world of emotional expression, Shakespeare's sonnets and the video game Doom each has its unique place.

megabyte (MB)   1,000,000 bytes. A thousand **kilobytes.**

megahertz (Mhz)   A million cycles per second.

metropolitan area network (MAN)   A data communication network fitted to a single urban region, theoretically able to promote data-sharing and service integration in an area.

Mhz   See **megahertz.**

MIB   See **medical information bus.**

microcomputer   A small computer based on a single-chip processor, such as a **PC.**

microprocessor   A computer-on-a-chip.

Microsoft   The company that was put on the map when IBM adopted its operating system, **DOS,** to install on its highly popular personal computers in 1980. Today **Windows,** DOS's **GUI** descendant, runs over 90 percent of the personal computers on the planet. Microsoft has big stakes in nearly every niche of the electronics world.

middleware   See **interface engine.**

millennium bug   Back before silicon wafers had become a commodity item and processing power was still the slow step in computer performance, programmers were motivated to write routines that were as spare as possible because leaner was faster and storage was expensive. One ubiquitous convention was to drop off the first two digits for the year in every date. Then it dawned on the computer world that the year 2000, represented as "00," might also be interpreted to mean 1900. Computers hate ambiguity. This one lurks in the hardware and software of millions of computers and other devices, promising to wreak widespread havoc for the unprepared as the clock ticks from 12/31/99 to 1/1/00. Based on predictions from some quarters of severe chaos resulting from the simultaneous failure of multiple computers that run the modern world's life-support systems, the millennium bug has given a real boost to the survivalist industry.

MIME   See **multipurpose Internet mail extension.**

minicomputer   One step down in computing power from a **mainframe.**

mirroring   A security procedure whereby a computer interposes itself between an internal user and the Internet. That computer creates an electronic image of the external server, filtering out all undesirable or potentially dangerous messages. The internal user then communicates with the network's own mirror site. Also a synonym for **duplexing,** meaning to run a backup computer identical to the primary computer to take over in case the primary device fails.

mission critical   Information which is top-priority for doing business.

modem   Short for "modulator-demodulator." A modem transforms digital to analog data for transmission along conventional phone lines, and then back to digital at the other end. Modems make the hisses, squeals, and pops that you hear when you accidentally pick up the phone receiver during transmission of a fax.

module   A set of software code that can be plugged in, as a whole, to accomplish a specific task in a larger program.

monitor   An electronic video display screen. Used to translate the output of everything from broadcast television to MRI scanners into visual images.

Moore's Law   After Gordon Moore, prior CEO of **Intel,** who observed in 1965 that the random access memory capacity of silicon computer chips that can be embedded in one square-inch doubled every eighteen months. This has held approximately true ever since, reflecting a several millionfold increase in memory on a single chip in about thirty-five years, a technological achievement without parallel in human history. Sooner or later chip design will irremediably bump up against the limits of physical laws, but we don't seem to be there yet.

motherboard   The card, usually made of fiberglass, which contains the **central processing unit** of a computer.

mouse   A computer input device first designed by engineers at Xerox. Movements of this hand-held device on its pad are reflected by a cursor on the computer screen. It can thus be used to draw or to issue commands.

Moving Picture Experts Group (MPEG)   Standards for compression and storage of motion video.

MPEG   See **Moving Picture Experts Group.**

multimedia   Combining more than one communication medium. Electronics has greatly enhanced the spectrum of possibilities, allowing communicators to construct messages using video, audio, still photos, text, music, branching logic structures, etc. Novel multimedia combinations may become media in their own right, much as audio and video have together become movies.

multiplexing   The next step after **duplexing.** A technology which allows multiple messages to be sent down the same channel simultaneously and sorted out at the receiving end.

multipurpose Internet mail extension (MIME)   A standard format for files that are attached to E-mail messages.

multitasking   The ability of a computer to run two or more programs simultaneously.

narrowband network   An electronic network connected by low bandwidth means, such as twisted pairs, that carries up to 64 Kbps.

National Committee for Quality Assurance (NCQA)   A private organization that assesses and reports the quality of managed care plans to assist purchasers and consumers with informed choice.

National Information Infrastructure (NII)   This is the formal name for the "information superhighway," the high-speed backbone of the Internet.

National Institute for Standards and Technology (NIST)   A branch of the U.S. Department of Commerce which awards grants for development of new technology, including technology in healthcare.

National Library of Medicine (NLM)   The world's largest medical library, maintained by the National Institutes of Health, has over five million holdings, most of them accessible via the **World Wide Web.**

National Provider Identifier (NPI)   System slated to replace the **UPIN.**

National Television Systems Committee (NTSC)   The U.S. standard for broadcast television, first adopted in 1953 for black-and-white.

natural language processing   The ability of an electronic system to analyze text-strings to some level of meaning, allowing for automatic coding, classifying, and analysis.

NCQA   See **National Council on Quality Assurance.**

netiquette   The (unwritten) rules for mannerly communication on the Internet.

Netscape   Founded in 1994, purchased by America Online in 1999, and already with a market capitalization in the billions, Netscape has built its fortune on Netscape Navigator, the most popular Internet **browser.** The big battle in browsers is between Navigator and Microsoft's Explorer, a battle that is being played out in the marketplace, in cyberspace, and in federal court.

network A group of data processing devices connected together so they may communicate with one another. A network may be more powerful and versatile (and also more hassle) than could be predicted by the sum of its parts.

network analyzer Security software that monitors network traffic for suspicious activity. Also called a **sniffer.**

network computer See **thin client.**

neural network An approach to **artificial intelligence** that uses a type of software designed to mimic the biological nervous system. It learns by adjusting the strength of the association between electronic constructs, much as the likelihood of signals passing between adjacent neurons changes as animals learn by experience. Neural networks have been put to use in decision support and pattern recognition.

newsgroup A discussion group on a specific topic resident on the Internet, maintained on a network or **bulletin board.**

Next Generation Internet (NGI) See **Internet 2.**

NGI See **Next Generation Internet.**

NII See **National Information Infrastructure.**

Nike net Slang for a situation in which messages are carried by hand, including by floppy disk, from person to person in the absence of an electronic network. Literally, you put on your Nikes and walk the message over to the recipient.

NIST See **National Institute for Standards and Technology.**

NLM See **National Library of Medicine.**

node Each device connected to a network is a node which sends and/or receives signals.

NPI See **National Provider Identifier.**

NTSC See **National Television Systems Committee.**

object-oriented technology A way of writing software that uses objects as building blocks. Objects are data stored along with **applets** which provide instructions on what to do with the data, as compared with segregating data and program files in traditional software. Object-oriented programming is supposed to be more efficient than conventional programming because of the ease with which objects may be assembled together.

OCR See **optical character recognition.**

OLTP See **on-line transaction processing.**

on-line/off-line To be on-line is to be actively connected to the network. Work may also be done off-line, then transmitted in batches.

on-line transaction processing (OLTP) The electronic frontline for many business functions in which work, such as patient registration, is done in real-time while connected to the network. Order entry is another common OLTP function of healthcare information systems.

open system   Software which easily admits additions and modifications. The code used in writing it must be available to the programmers who want to work on it.

open systems interconnection (OSI)   A standard that provides a framework for implementing communication protocols in seven layers.

operating system   Alan Turing and John von Neuman demonstrated, when they developed the theory of universal computing device in the 1940s and '50s, that a machine could be made to perform any logical task given the right instructions (software). The operating system tells a universal computing device (computer) what kind of device to be. It specifies how each of the components— processor, memory, input and output, storage devices, etc.—will function and how it will communicate with the other components. Application software, which does the actual work, sits atop the operating system. **DOS, Windows, Macintosh, Linux,** and **UNIX** are operating systems.

optical character recognition (OCR)   Unlike the fax, which records and transmits printed text as images, this process uses specialized hardware and software to transform it to digital form. Once scanned as character code into a computer by an OCR device, text gains all the benefits of being digital, including searchability and compressability.

OSI   See **open systems interconnection.**

outcomes research   The ultimate goal for the use of aggregate patient data by any healthcare system. It correlates what was done to patients with how (if at all) their health was affected by the care. Outcomes may be measured in years-of-life saved, function, comfort, dollars, satisfaction, or a host of other factors. Good management of individual patients and of healthcare organizations overall will come to depend heavily on outcomes research.

packet   A bundle of data ready for transmission.

packet switching   Sending addressed **packet**s of data through a network.

PACS   See **picture archiving and communication system.**

palmtop   The next step down in size and computing power from a notebook computer. Typically, a palmtop is used in the field to carry and record data. It should fit in a clothes pocket, at least a large one. Most palmtops can exchange information and software with bigger machines.

paradigm shift   Term coined by Thomas Kuhn in his 1970 classic *The Structure of Scientific Revolutions* to describe the discontinuity that occurs when one scientific world view is replaced by another, such as when the heliocentric model replaced the geocentric solar system. The term has been adopted by management gurus as part of their routine to get members of organizations to think creatively.

password   The code which allows a user access to a system or set of data. It is the first step in security.

PBX See **private branch exchange.**

PC See **personal computer.**

PCMCIA See **personal computer memory card/international association.**

PDA See **personal digital assistant.**

Pentium The currently reigning processor for desktop computers, built by **Intel** Corporation. There are multiple versions of Pentium chips available at a wide range of power, clock speed, and price.

performance Measured speed and reliability of a system or device performing a specific task. See **benchmarking.**

peripheral devices The machines connected to a computer, such as monitors, modems, printers, and scanners.

personal computer (PC) Originally known as a microcomputer. A smallish machine that can stand alone for use by one person at a time. PCs that are tied into a network can also work cooperatively.

personal computer memory card/international association (PCMCIA) A credit-card sized computer board which can be plugged into special slots on a PC to add a fax/modem, additional memory, video and graphics capabilities, or network connectivity.

personal digital assistant (PDA) A palmtop-size device that holds personally useful information such as address and date books, account records, documents, etc. Following the principle of **convergence,** many PDAs now also serve as modems, phones, and pagers.

petabyte (PB) 1,000,000,000,000 bytes. A thousand **terabytes.**

photonics The science of using photons to do computing and communicating. Photons are faster and capable of providing much higher bandwidth to photonic devices than electrons provide to electronic devices. This field is in its infancy.

picture archiving and communication system (PACS) A PACS acquires, stores, accesses, and displays images in digital format. An important part of any digital radiology system.

picture-in-picture (PIP) A common feature in video conferencing that allows views from more than one camera to be displayed on one monitor. For example, the main video display may be of a presenter with a PIP of a questioner from the audience.

PIP See **picture-in-picture.**

pixel The smallest element in a video display. A pixel is uniquely specified by a group of numbers that locate it on the screen and indicate its brightness and color. The more pixels per unit of area, the higher the resolution.

plain-old telephone service (POTS) A slightly tongue-in-cheek description of the low bandwidth means by which most of us are connected to the planet's nervous system. See **last mile problem.**

platform Name for the operating system plus machine. Choosing a platform is the first step towards building any electronic system.

plug-and-play A rarely-met ideal for an electronic system indicating that the user merely has to plug it in, turn it on, and start to use it. It is highly unusual for a system of any complexity to require no setup or training. **Turnkey system** is a synonym.

point of presence (POP) Any place that a health system reaches is a point of presence. In computer terms, the sum of points of presence describes the total potential **nodes** of a system.

POP See **point of presence** and **post office protocol.**

port Just as in transportation of materials, in the world of electronics a port is a place where things—in this case messages—begin and end their journeys. It is the connecting point between machines, where cables plug in and where radio, infrared, and other types of signals are received. Synonym: "portal."

postmodernism A term coined by followers of the French philosopher, Michel Foucault, to describe the literary movement that comes after and in reaction to modernism. In contrast to its predecessor, postmodernist thought and art are ornamented, eclectic, inductive, decentralized, mutable, and nondeterministic. Multimedia, audio sampling, and hypertext—all made possible by computers—are typical techniques of the postmodern aesthetic.

post office protocol (POP) A routine for storing mail on servers until it is picked up by the addressees.

POTS See **plain-old telephone service.**

practice guidelines Parameters, hopefully incorporating the latest knowledge and best understanding of a disease process, that serve to guide practitioners towards the best, most efficient treatment decisions. In an effort to find terms to assuage physicians who are wary of what they fear is "cookbook medicine," they are also called "practice parameters" and "pathways."

practitioner A professional who delivers care directly to patients. The term is usually reserved for those with more autonomy such as nurse practitioners, physical therapists, physicians, physician assistants, dentists, etc. Sometimes called a **provider,** a term which the Joint Commission for Accreditation of Healthcare Organizations reserves for organizations.

printer The device which outputs computer data onto paper as "hard copy."

private branch exchange (PBX) The "switchboard" which routes phone calls between devices within a network and between the network and outside.

process management Applying quantitative quality control techniques to meeting quality, cost, and productivity goals.

programming language The conventions that human programmers use to write instructions for machines. Programming language codes must be translated by a **compiler** into **machine language,** which is always in binary code.

protocol   In the context of electronic communications, the software conventions that allow one machine to "talk" to another.

provider   An organization which provides healthcare, such as a hospital, clinic, integrated delivery system, or health plan. Sometimes used synonymously for **practitioner.**

proxy server   An **http** engine which mediates communication between nodes within a network to outside sites, on the other side of the **firewall.** See **mirroring.**

public-key encryption   Mathematical algorithms which allow messages to be encoded, transmitted securely, and authenticated without resorting to the weak link of a common secret key that must be maintained by both sender and receiver.

pull technology   Receivers decide what information they want and go after it. Web surfing, because it is initiated by the receiver, is a pull technology.

push technology   The networking equivalent of broadcasting, ie., sending messages which have not been individually requested by the receiver. Listservs, which initiate the distribution of E-mail messages, are push technology.

QoS   See **quality of service.**

quality of service (QoS)   Where network access and speed of data transmission are critical, users may enter into QoS contracts with communication companies that provide specific guarantees of rates of data delivery.

radio frequency   Radio frequency is a wireless communication modality that can be used to provide connectivity between devices. Unlike cellular technology, these signals do not have the potential to disrupt electronic medical equipment.

RAM   See **random access memory.**

random access memory (RAM)   Sort of a notepad in a computer's processor where active data and parts of programs are stored for immediate use. RAM is fast and volatile. In general, the more RAM a computer has the faster it can do things and the more things it can do simultaneously.

RAS   See **reliability, availability, serviceability.**

raster graphics   Images built on a grid, a point at a time, with **pixels.** Compare to **vector graphics.**

RBOC   See **Regional Bell Operating Company.**

real-time   Viewing, processing, or transmitting something in real-time is to do it within a fraction of a second of when it is occurring, as opposed to storing it for later processing and use. Compare to **store-and-forward.**

receiver operating characteristic (ROC)   The human part of any electronic system which determines, ultimately, how well it works. For example, one can describe precisely just how fine a distinction in colors and textures of skin lesions a video transmission system can record and display. But it is the ROC of the doctor at the receiving end which ultimately determines whether the system is any good for distinguishing a malignant from a benign lesion.

red green blue (RGB)   The code that controls the cathode ray tube in color video monitors.

redundancy   Because of the critical functions which they perform, many medical systems need to be fault tolerant. Redundancy, duplicating some or all of critical systems so as to provide backup, is one of the most important strategies for building in fault tolerance. See **mirroring.**

re-engineering   A management term for re-designing work processes. In order to best realize efficiency gains, re-engineering must sometimes go hand-in-hand with automation instead of just automating existing suboptimal practices.

Regional Bell Operating Company (RBOC)   Pronounced "R-Bock," these "Baby Bells" resulted from the breakup of AT&T in the 1980s. With deregulation removing their restrictions from playing outside their original regions, the RBOCs have fast become major forces in national and international telecommunications markets.

relational database   A structured way of storing data in a computer in two-dimensional tables. Relational databases allow easy comparison of data and updating of different elements by tying them together. For example, changing a patient's street address in a relational database would cause the new address to appear on every report about and mailing to that patient and could be designed to automatically change the zip code too.

release   Successful software is constantly evolving and improving. Each updated version is called a release. These are usually labeled in some sort of numerical order, e.g., version 7.3 might replace version 7.2, both of which are supplanted later by version 8.0.

reliability, availability, serviceability (RAS)   The opposite of these measures is a good approximation of the costs and hassles of maintaining an electronic system.

remote computing   Allowing a client access to an organization's data processing center. Remote computing solutions can, by economies of scale provided by multiple users, give each user access to more computing power at less cost. Because information resides on one computer, remote computing can also facilitate data consolidation and analysis.

resolution   Resolution is a measure of how fine the detail an imaging system can display. Resolution and **ROC** together are the key determinants of the utility of a medical imaging system.

resolver   A software program which untangles ambiguities in data. Patient identification resolvers are key components in **electronic medical records** systems.

RGB   See **red green blue.**

ring topology   A pattern of network connections where data are passed around from machine to machine in a closed circle. **Ethernet** is the best-known exploiter of this topology.

robotics   The branch of informatics that designs and deploys electronic devices to do actual physical work. Robots vary enormously in their sophistication and capabilities, from simple motor-driven actuators to intelligent sensing device-laden multipurpose machines. The word "robot" was coined in 1920 by Karel Capek, a Czech dramatist.

robust   A robust system is one that consistently functions well, with little down time.

ROC   See **receiver operating characteristic.**

rollabout unit   A teleconferencing or telemedicine unit which contains cameras, **codec, monitor,** and other devices and can be rolled from room to room. Compare to **room unit** and **set-top system.**

room unit   A fixed teleconferencing or telemedicine unit. Compare to **rollabout unit** and **set-top system.**

router   A communications computer that sorts and relays messages over a network.

S&F   See **store-and-forward.**

scalability   A critical characteristic to consider when selecting a computer system. Scalability means that the system has the potential to grow to meet increasing needs, rather than becoming obsolete and having to be replaced.

scanning   Converting an analog document, picture, X ray, etc. into a digital replica which can be stored, processed, and accessed by a computer.

search engine   Software that catalogues Internet sites and their content and then serves as an index. The biggest search engines function nearly autonomously, browsing the web and bringing back information for the index. Yahoo, Lycos, Excite, AltaVista, InfoSeek, and HotBot are some of the most popular engines. Each uses different techniques to organize information and searches. See **gateway.**

self-organizing systems   This concept was first elucidated by Ilya Prigogine, the Nobel prizewinning Belgian physicist who investigated the mathematics of how more complex biological systems grow out of simpler systems in the course of evolution. These same principles provide important insights when applied to the world of computers and electronic communications.

server   A computer in a network which provides connections, data, and software to other computers, called **clients.**

set-top system   A **dial-up** videoconferencing system, including camera and **codec,** that are paired with ordinary televisions and computer video monitors. Compare to **room unit** and **rollabout unit.**

shareware Software placed into the public domain where it is available for free or a very low fee.

simple mail transfer protocol (SMTP) The electronic rules by which E-mail is exchanged between machines.

simulation Using a digital model of a system based upon its structure and properties, a computer can calculate how that system will perform. It is generally much less costly to try out processes and products by simulation, even before they are ever constructed, than to test them in the real world.

simulator sickness Nausea, vertigo, and disorientation induced by disrupting normal feedback among eyes, inner ear, and brain with **virtual reality** gear.

small computer system interface (SCSI) A fast variety of PC **port** used to attach to peripheral devices. Pronounced "scuzzy."

smart card A device which contains up to 8,000 characters, compared to the 72 which can be encoded onto the magnetic strip of a similarly-sized credit card. In the medical field smart cards are being used today to store data such as insurance information, health problems, allergy and drug lists, and electro-cardiograms in a completely portable format that stays with patients everywhere (as long as you don't lose your wallet or purse). The problem, of course, is that most healthcare sites have not adopted smart card technology and so cannot read the data.

SMTP See **simple mail transfer protocol.**

snail mail U.S. Postal Service or other physical transport medium for messages. Compared to the light speed of **E-mail.**

sniffer See **network analyzer.**

SNOMED See **systematized nomenclature for human and veterinary medicine.**

socket The combination of an **IP address** and a **port** number. The exact place where one machine is "plugged into" another while they are communicating.

software The instructions which run a machine (**hardware**).

sound card A micro-processor that can sample, record, and store analog sounds in digital format.

source code After a software program is created it is usually put through a process called compiling which translates the programmer's language into **machine language.** Compiling squeezes out a good deal of the redundancy and other features which make the program intelligible to the programmer but slow for the computer. Unfortunately, this is a one-way function; uncompiling a program is like getting the toothpaste back into the tube. The source code is the original humanly intelligible program, which is where a programmer goes to edit, fix, and update a program. It also contains the proprietary secrets of the software. Negotiating access to source code is an important piece of many computer deals. **Open systems** publish their source code. Closed systems don't.

spam   Unsolicited, unwanted E-mail. From a Monty Python routine, set in a restaurant, where "spam" is the only item on the menu and repeated to the point of nausea. A breach of **netiquette,** spamming may invite **flaming.**

speech recognition   One of the biggest disappointments in computer science is that by 2001 we will not have a computer that understands human speech like HAL did in the science fiction movie named after that year. Automating the job that transcriptionists do has turned out to be a much more difficult task than anticipated. Speech recognition software has found use in some limited medical areas with narrower vocabularies and more standardized formats such as for radiology interpretation reports.

spooling   When there is a bottleneck in processing, such as output to a slow printer, the computer resorts to spooling the pending jobs, which means putting the data in a queue to wait their turn for processing. Meanwhile, the computer can perform other tasks.

SQL   See **structured query language.**

standard   An agreed-upon way of doing something with hardware or software. Standards may be mandated by authoritative groups such as the **IEEE** or **ISO,** or they may be determined by the marketplace. Lack of standards which guarantee **interoperability** has been one of the greatest impediments to development of medical information systems.

star topology   A network architecture in which a server central to the network maintains an individual connection to each of the other nodes. Synonym: **hub-and-spoke.**

store-and-forward (S&F)   This feature liberates telemedicine practitioners from constraints placed by time. It allows data to be accessed, reviewed, and acted upon at a time and place remote from the patient encounter. **E-mail** is an S&F system.

structured query language (SQL)   The standard language for extracting information from a **relational database.**

Sun Microsystems   This company made its fortune producing computer workstations, high-power PCs used by scientists, animators, and others with heavy duty data processing needs. Lately it has staked its fortune on leveraging **Java,** its popular applet-based language most useful for Internet applications, along with strategic investments in Internet-based businesses.

switch   A device which determines the path of electrical impulses. Switches are at the heart of every computer and communications network.

switched line   A telecommunications connection that is made (and charged for) as it is needed. Compare to **leased line.**

sys admin   See **system administrator.**

sysop   See **system administrator.**

system administrator (sys admin or sysop)   The boss of a network who is responsible for keeping it functional. An important person to be on the good side of.

system analyst An information systems professional who specializes in matching system design to desired function.

systematized nomenclature for human and veterinary medicine (SNOMED) A standardized vocabulary developed by the College of American Pathologists. Considered by some experts as the best starting point for developing a standardized vocabulary for **computer-based patient records.**

T1 Telephone connection capable of carrying 1.544 Mbps. The equivalent of twenty-four twisted pairs.

T3 Telephone connection capable of carrying 44.74 Mbps.

TATRC See **Telemedicine and Advanced Technology Research Center.**

TB See **terabyte.**

TCP/IP See **transmission control protocol/internet protocol.**

technical support See **maintainence.**

technology The application of scientific methods to achieve a practical purpose.

telco A company that provides phone service.

telehealth See **telemedicine.**

telemedicine The combined use of telecommunications and computer technologies to improve efficiency and effectiveness of healthcare services by liberating caregivers from traditional constraints of place and time and by empowering consumers to make informed choices in a competitive marketplace.

Telemedicine and Advanced Technology Research Center (TATRC) A tri-forces (Army, Navy, and Air Force) command located on the military base at Ft. Detrick in Frederick, Maryland. Many of the systems used in telemedicine were designed and developed at TATRC.

telementoring Distant supervision of training via electronic means.

telepresence The network-enabled ability of a person in one place to participate in activity at another location, as in telepresence surgery, where a surgeon who is not physically present in an operating room can remotely control surgical equipment inserted by a technician who is present with the patient.

teleproctoring An extension of **telementoring,** where performance is documented for privileging and other purposes.

teleradiology A system for providing diagnostic imaging studies at a site distant from where they were performed using images transmitted by electronic means.

terabyte (TB) 1,000,000,000 bytes. A thousand **gigabytes.**

thin client A computer of limited capacity that receives some of the data and software that it needs from a **server** as it needs it. The "thinnest client" contains virtually no individual processing power and receives its programs as it needs them from a server.

thumbnails Miniature, low-resolution images that can download quickly for review and be used for selecting which images to view at higher resolution.

tiered architecture A way of structuring a network for efficiency so that different layers of machines work with different layers of data. This way processing power can be best matched to data needs at each level.

tool-based solution Provision of a software "tool set" which allows users to customize a system to their needs rather than being stuck with unmodifiable (hard-coded) software.

topology The most general description of connections in a network. **Ring, bus,** and **star** are three common topologies, each with its own strengths and weaknesses.

transmission control protocol/Internet protocol (TCP/IP) These are the basic rules for getting computers to communicate in the language of the **Internet.** They tell computers how to identify themselves, address, structure, and acknowledge messages. They are also the guiding principles of every **intranet** and **extranet.**

transmission rate How fast data can be moved from one point to another is the transmission rate of that part of the system. Synonymous with **bandwidth.**

turnkey system See **plug-and-play.**

twisted pair The copper wires by which most of us are connected to the public phone network. At best, a modem can transmit data on a twisted pair at the rate of 56 Kbps.

UMLS See **Unified Medical Language System.**

Unified Medical Language System (UMLS) An ongoing project by the **National Library of Medicine** to expand and coordinate the terminology used in medical databases.

uninterrupted power supply (UPS) An emergency power source that is supposed to keep a system from crashing in the event of loss of electrical power. The time it functions is determined by the capacity of the storage batteries or generator, but should be at least long enough to shut down the system in an orderly way that avoids data loss.

universal patient identifier (UPI) The first step in creating any electronic patient record. It is the code number, unique to each individual, under which all patient-specific medical information is filed. By using the UPI, all the data about patients could be brought together from disparate sources to present a comprehensive view of their experience. See **master patient index** and **resolver.**

universal physician provider number (UPIN) The current system, rolled out in 1985, by which the U.S. Health Care Financing Administration identifies all physicians who bill services under Medicare.

universal resource locator (URL)   **World Wide Web** address. Typically in the form http://www.sitename.domain. See **domain.**

Unix   An operating system developed by Bell Laboratories and released in 1969, designed to run on devices ranging from personal computers to mainframes. Unix's ability to cross platforms and reliability placed it at the heart of most communication systems, where it still resides today. Multiple versions of Unix have evolved.

UPI   See **universal patient identifier.**

UPIN   See **universal physician provider number.**

upload   To send data from a computer. The opposite of **download.**

UPS   See **uninterrupted power supply.**

URL   See **universal resource locator.**

Usenet   A giant electronic bulletin board in cyberspace where thousands of **newsgroups** post messages and carry on conversations on the Internet.

user   A human who interacts with an information system. Sometimes called "grayware" for gray matter.

vaporware   When they are making their sales pitch, software vendors often promise that certain features are being developed and will be rolled out soon. All too often these promised features fail to materialize.

vector graphics   A way of representing computer displays mathematically employing vectors. Especially valuable for doing animation because, unlike **raster** images, vector images can be moved, resized, and recolored without losing their shape.

video conference   A meeting in **cyberspace** that employs interactive video.

video on demand (VoD)   The ability to provide instantaneous access to remotely stored video. Limitations of bandwidth and video servers make this technology very expensive. Most prevalent installations are currently used for entertainment of hotel guests.

videophone   Small audio-video units which work over **POTS** or **ISDN** connections and are not dependent on external computers or other larger systems. See **set-top system.**

virtual integrated delivery system   Tying together, by electronic technology, separate practices and institutions in a market so that they function as an integrated system. As yet, an unrealized concept.

virtual private network (VPN)   See **extranet.**

virtual reality   A multimedia representation that, by way of its persuasiveness or power, acquires the status of an alternative constructed reality. Flight simulators used for pilot training, for example, strive to be virtual reality devices. A lot of money and a lot of science fiction (see, for example the Holodeck on "Star Trek, The New Generation") are devoted to the potential of electronically constructed virtual realities.

virus Just as its biological cousins live by taking over the machinery of a healthy organism, a software virus survives by insinuating itself into a "healthy" machine's software codes, where it may quietly coexist, reproduce, jump to other machines, and sometimes wreak havoc on every system it touches.

VoD See **video on demand.**

voice recognition See **speech recognition.**

VPN See **extranet.**

W3C See **World Wide Web Consortium.**

WAN See **wide area network.**

Web See **World Wide Web.**

Web-enabled This refers to a computer that is capable of following World Wide Web protocols, whether on the Internet or an intranet.

Webmaster A person who creates or manages a **Website.**

Website A **node** on the **World Wide Web,** identified by a **URL.**

wetware Biological computing systems, particularly brains.

what you see is what you get (WYSIWYG) A video display feature which says that what shows up on the screen is close to what the document will look like when printed. Pronounced "wissywig."

whiteboard A peripheral device to video conferencing that works like a communal doodle pad for brainstorming sessions. Also good for passing messages to try to fix the audio portion when it doesn't work.

wide area network (WAN) A data network confined within an enterprise that extends far beyond a local area, such as between cities, states, and countries. Compare to **LAN** and **MAN.**

wideband network Somewhere between **narrowband**'s 64 Kbps and **broadband**'s 1.5 Mbps transmission rates.

Windows (3.1, '95, NT, '97) **Microsoft**'s omnipresent operating system, a **GUI** which replaced (actually was written on top of) **DOS,** its initial megahit system. There are several versions. Windows '98 is currently the latest.

wired Slang to describe somebody who is connected to the Internet. Among technophiles "wired" implies a slew of knowledge about, facility with, and positive attitudes towards electronic technology. Contrast to **Luddite.**

wireless Connected electronically via **radio frequency, Ir,** or other waves that do not mandate a physical link between machines.

workstation A beefed up **PC.**

World Wide Web (WWW) The hypertext-based part of the Internet, introduced in 1990 by Tim Berners-Lee who developed the first Web browser and server at CERN, the European nuclear physics research organization. Because of its ease of use and ability to incorporate multimedia, the WWW has made the Internet a popular phenomenon.

World Wide Web Consortium (W3C)   The international consortium that develops standards for the Web.

WWW   See **World Wide Web.**

WYSIWYG   See **what you see is what you get.**

XML   See **eXtensible Markup Language.**

Y2K   See **millennium bug.**

Year 2000 (Y2K)   See **millennium bug.**

INDEX

A

Access, 79
  real-time, 33
Acupuncture, 32
AI. *See* Artificial intelligence
AIDS. *See* Autoimmune
  deficiency syndrome
Allen, Ace, M.D., 44–45
American Telemedicine
  Association (ATA), 163
    health provider criteria,
      178–179
    patient criteria, 177–178
    technology criteria, 179
    tele-homecare clinical
      guidelines, 177–179
Analysis, remote of ICU data,
  132–133
Anesthesia, 62–63
Antibiotics, 71–72
Artificial intelligence (AI), 93
Association of Telemedicine
  Service Providers (ATSP), 89,
  163
ATA. *See* American Telemedicine
  Association
ATM. *See* Automated teller
  machines
ATSP. *See* Association of
  Telemedicine Service Providers
Authentication, 171
Authorization, 171–172
Autoimmune deficiency
  syndrome (AIDS), 73
Automated teller machines
  (ATM), 131

B

Baby pictures, 42–43
Bacteriology, 66
Balanced Budget Act (1997), 161
Bandwith, 140–142
Behavioral teletherapy for
  soldiers, 128–129
Boolean algebra, 185
Branding, 184

C

Cable television, 40
Caputo, Michael, 54–55
CHESS. *See* Comprehensive
  Health Enhancement Support
  Systems
Claims review process, 100
Clayton Antitrust Act (1914),
  69
Clinical practice guidelines
  (CPG), 176–177
Clinical protocols, 33
CME. *See* Continuing medical
  education
Commercial-off-the-shelf (COTS)
  devices, 171
  systems, 127, 151
Communications, 39
  images, 37–38
  satellites, 40
Community health information,
  170–171
Compliance, 96
Comprehensive dental care,
  46–47

ABOUT THE AUTHORS

Dr. Jeff Bauer is one of the country's most respected futurists and medical economists. He has a Ph.D. in medical economics and has written over 60 articles and books on healthcare delivery, including *Not What the Doctor Ordered* (revised edition: McGraw-Hill, 1998) and *Statistical Analysis for Decision Makers in Healthcare* (McGraw-Hill, 1996). He speaks frequently to national audiences about the future of healthcare and is quoted often in the healthcare press. Dr. Bauer has been a professor at the medical schools of the University of Colorado and the University of Wisconsin-Madison, and he is the Senior Fellow for health policy studies at the Center for the New West in Denver, Colorado.

Dr. Marc Ringel is a family practice physician in rural Colorado who also works as a medical education consultant and medical director for a long-term care facility. When Dr. Ringel is not busy with his professional duties, he serves as a regular commentator on the APR radio show "Marketplace," addressing issues relating to rural practice and medical information technology. Dr. Ringel has published numerous articles and items in journals such as *Postgraduate Medicine,* the *Journal of the MGMA,* and *Emergency Medicine,* and has contributed chapters to such clinical references as the *Saunders Manual of Medical Practice.*